D0276949

Healthcare Professionals as Witnesses to the Court

Healthcare Professionals as Witnesses to the Court

Colin J. Holburn FFAEM FRCS(Ed)
Consultant in Accident & Emergency Medicine
Sandwell General Hospital
West Midlands

Catherine Bond MA(Cantab) PGCE FRSA
Solicitor
Bond Solon Training
London

Mark Solon MSc FRSA
Solicitor
Bond Solon Training
London

Suzanne Burn LLB LLM
Solicitor
Legal Training Consultant
Deputy District Judge
London

GREENWICH MEDICAL MEDIA LTD
137 Euston Road
London
NW1 2AA

ISBN 1 900 151 227

First Published 2000

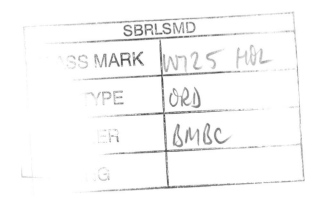

Typeset by Saxon Graphics Ltd, Derby

Printed in Great Britain by
The Alden Group, Oxford

Visit our website at
www.greenwich-medical.co.uk

CONTENTS

Dedications

For Paula and the boys, thanks for the support.

C.H.

For my mother and my father, with love and for my second child, as yet unborn, in excited anticipation

C.B.

For my father

M.S.

For David – my inspiration

S.B.

PREFACE

This book is designed not as an academic tome on the legal system in England and Wales but a practical guide for health care professionals in their involvement in the system. It is not intended as a substitute for attending training in the relevant knowledge and skills.

Because of the layout of the book certain advice is of necessity repeated in order to avoid the reader having to cross refer to other parts of the book.

We hope that this makes the book more readable for a professional asked to engage in a particular activity at one time. It does not mean that the book cannot or should not be read in its entirety. As experts and lawyers are of both sexes, we have freely used both the masculine and feminine pronouns. Each obviously includes the other. The law is stated as at 1 July 1999.

C.H.
C.B.
M.S.
S.B.

July 1999

Introduction to the English Legal System

This chapter sets out a brief introduction to the English legal system in order to put the role of the health care professional as witness into context. The introduction is simplified to aid understanding. The principles are expanded in later chapters.

What is the adversarial system?

In general, courts in England and Wales have an adversarial system. Two parties (or perhaps more) come before the court, usually represented by their lawyers. Their version of events is in dispute. The court must find out what happened, taking into account evidence of fact and expert opinion.

With the permission of the court each party is entitled to call its own oral evidence. It also has the opportunity to cross-examine, by means of critical questions, the evidence of its opponent's witnesses. The court will also look at other evidence such as documentary evidence. Each side will often have its own expert witness.

What is the difference between criminal and civil cases?

In the English legal system there are two types of case, criminal and civil. Criminal cases occur when the Crown or state alleges that a crime has been committed. The person accused of the crime, the defendant, is generally prosecuted by the Crown Prosecution Service. The defendant is deemed innocent until proven guilty beyond reasonable doubt. Criminal trials are heard either at a Magistrates Court or a Crown Court. In the latter case there will be a jury.

In civil cases, individuals or corporate organisations take other individuals or organisations to court where there is a dispute between them which cannot be resolved by other means. Here the party bringing the claim is called the claimant. It has to prove its case on a balance of probabilities, i.e. what the claimant suggests happened is more likely to have happened than not.

Civil cases are tried either at the County Court or the High Court. There is no jury except in cases of defamation and in other very limited circumstances. Healthcare practitioners may be required in many types of civil claim, including personal injury cases, professional negligence and fatal accident cases.

Who is who in the legal profession?

Solicitors

Solicitors are responsible for advising the client, preparing documents and evidence for court and negotiating settlement of the case. They handle the planning, tactics and running of the case and instruct experts and, when necessary, barristers. Solicitors have rights of audience (i.e. the right to speak) in the County Court and sometimes in the High Court.

Barristers

Barristers are, sometimes, instructed by solicitors to represent the client in court and have rights of audience in all the courts. They specialise in advocacy.

But they may also be asked by solicitors to advise or draft documents for court especially in the more complex or high value cases and/or when difficult or new questions of law are involved.

Leading counsel

Leading counsel, sometimes referred to as a QC or a silk, is a senior barrister with usually at least twenty years experience as a barrister.

Junior counsel

This is a term used to describe a barrister who is not a leading counsel.

What does the County Court do?

The County Court is one of the two types of civil court where cases are commenced and trials held (the other being the High Court). Proceedings in respect of personal injury litigation must be commenced in the County Court unless the value of the action is £50,000 or more (in which case proceedings may be started in the High Court). However, there is no limit to the damages that can be awarded in the County Court.

Proceedings for other types of litigation must be started in the County Court unless the value of the action is £15,000 or more (before 26 April 1999 the amount was £5,000).

The County Court also deals with the majority of family disputes (divorce, money settlements and children) and most landlord and tenant actions (both housing and business premises).

The District Judge

District Judges manage the pre-trial work of most claims in the County Court and hear the trials of cases up to £15,000 in value. Most District Judges come from the solicitors' profession. A District Judge is addressed as 'Sir' or 'Madam'.

Circuit Judge/Recorder/Assistant Recorder

These judges usually try actions where the sum in issue is more than £15,000. They are addressed as *'Your Honour.'* Most Circuit Judges and Recorders come from the barristers' profession.

What does the High Court do?

The High Court has several divisions or departments as follows:

(i)   Queen's Bench Division including: negligence, personal injury, and contract disputes; (the Commercial Court which handles the more complex commercial disputes is part of the Queen's Bench Division).

(ii) Chancery Division including: trusts, probate, land disputes, partnership action.

(iii) Family Division: Matrimonial and Children Act cases.

(iv) The Specialist Divisions which include Admiralty, Companies Court, Patents Court and Construction and Technology Court.

A High Court hearing is usually presided over by one judge. He or she can be a Circuit Judge, a High Court judge or senior Q.C.

A High Court judge should be addressed as *'Your Lordship/Ladyship.'*

The 'Tracking System'

From 26 April 1999, when the Civil Procedure Rules 1998 came into force, all defended claims are allocated to one of three 'management tracks', in which different procedures, degrees of judicial control and costs rules are followed which are appropriate and proportionate to the amount in dispute and the complexity of the case. The Small Claims and Fast Tracks are part of the County Court: cases on the third track, the Multi track, may be 'managed' by District Judges in the County Court but usually are tried by Circuit or High Court judges.

The Small Claims track is the normal track for claims up to £5,000 (previously £3,000) except for personal injury and housing disrepair where the limit is £1,000. Hearings are informal before a District Judge. Strict rules of evidence do not apply and there are only limited rights of appeal.

The Fast Track is the normal track for claims with a value between £5,000 and £15,000 (personal injury and housing disrepair £1,000 to £15,000) where the issues in dispute are not complicated, and the trial can be heard in one day, usually without oral evidence from experts.

The Multi Track is the normal track for claims with a value over £15,000, or lower value claims which involve several parties or more complex issues of law, fact or evidence, and which require more judicial case management.

The Court decides to which track a case should be allocated, if and when it is defended: the parties are sent detailed questionnaires to complete (Allocation Questionnaires) which ask for information on the number of witnesses, whether expert evidence may be needed, whether there are any complicating factors and how long the trial may take.

The intention in the Civil Procedure Rules is to decide all Small Claims and Fast Track cases within 30 weeks of their allocation to a track: previously some of these lower value claims would take 1–2 years to reach trial.

Multi track cases will receive their own individual timetables but the aim is still to set as early a trial date as possible for the parties to work towards.

What does the Court of Appeal (Civil Division) do?

Appeals from a decision of a District Judge are usually heard by a Circuit Judge, and from a decision by a Circuit Judge are heard by a High Court Judge: effectively the case is reheard. Only the more complex or difficult appeals are heard by the Court of Appeal: in nearly all cases permission is needed from the judge hearing the trial or appeal in the previous court, or from the Court of Appeal itself.

The Court of Appeal does not retry the case but reviews the paperwork and listens to the legal argument.

Usually three judges 'sit' and the decision is by majority.

A Court of Appeal judge should be addressed as '*Your Lordship/Ladyship*'.

What does the House of Lords do?

The House of Lords only hears cases where there is a point of law that is of great public importance. It sits in the Committee rooms in the Houses of Parliament at Westminster.

Normally there are between three and seven (usually five) Lords of Appeal. Sometimes the Lord Chancellor will preside.

The correct form of address is '*Your Lordship/Ladyship.*'

Who are the parties to proceedings in the Civil Courts?

Litigation is between claimants and defendants.

The claimant

A claimant is an individual or organisation who starts a court action. Usually he believes that he has suffered a wrongful loss. For example, he may have been physically injured in a road traffic accident which he believes was the fault of another party or that he has been given negligent professional treatment in hospital. The claimant normally wishes to claim money from the person or organisation who he considers has caused the loss but who has, so far, refused to accept responsibility. The claimant brings a court action (sues) to obtain financial compensation in the form of damages from a defendant.

There are two things that the claimant has to prove to the Court:

(i) That the person being sued (the defendant) is responsible for having caused the injury, etc. This is known as liability;

(ii) That he has lost an amount of money mainly as a result of the defendant's actions (this is called 'quantum', a Latin word meaning amount).

The defendant

The defendant is the person or organisation from whom money is claimed. An example would be a motorist who has run over a pedestrian and injured him. The compensation is called damages. If the defendant loses in respect of liability, an order to pay damages will be made. The losing defendant is not 'guilty', but merely said to be liable to the claimant. The court passes judgment and will order the defendant to pay a specified amount of money.

Where the defendant is insured (for example, a motorist who causes an accident resulting in personal injury) the defence will usually be run by his insurance company.

In civil cases, what is the burden and standard of proof?

The legal burden

The burden of proving the claim lies with the party bringing the action, i.e. the claimant. So, if a claimant is alleging professional negligence, he or she must prove all the elements of the tort (civil wrong) of negligence as follows:

(i) That a duty of care existed between the claimant and the defendant.

(ii) That the defendant breached this duty of care.

(iii) That the breach caused the claimant loss/damage.

(iv) The amount of the loss/damage.

The standard of proof

In civil cases, the claimant is required to prove his case on a balance of probabilities. This is an easier burden than the 'beyond reasonable doubt' required in criminal cases. It means that the judge must be persuaded that the claimant's version of events is more likely than the defendant's to be true.

What is the procedure in civil cases?

Prior to starting civil cases

The first stage is for the potential claimant to decide whether he/she has a worthwhile case, whether the defendant will be able to pay, and whether the likely value of the claim is sufficient to justify the costs of investigating and proving it.

Recognising that litigation is often stressful, complex, expensive and can take some time, the reforms of the civil justice system brought into force in April 1999 through the Civil Procedure Rules 1998, encourage parties to a claim or dispute to regard "litigation as a last resort" and to try first to settle their differences by negotiation or other means.

In a typical personal injury case, the accident victim will seek advice from a solicitor, who will collect sufficient information to advise what might be done (e.g in a road traffic case the police report and statements from any eyewitnesses). A medical report from an appropriate doctor will also be required and sometimes advice or a report from other independent experts (e.g in a factory accident case from a health and safety expert).

The Civil Procedure Rules require parties to a dispute to work together to resolve it *before* starting a court action. Potential claimants are strongly encouraged to send to the potential defendant as soon as possible a detailed letter which sets out their version of the events, explains why it is felt the defendant is to blame and which gives an outline at least of the losses suffered. The defendant should be allowed a reasonable amount of time to investigate and reply before the claimant moves to the next stage – issuing proceedings.

If the defendant is willing to accept responsibility the parties should then discuss what other information is needed to settle the claim and try to do so by negotiation. If the defendant does not accept responsibility the parties should, nonetheless, continue to work together to prepare the case for court proceedings by sharing information – exchanging relevant paperwork, and discussing the other 'evidence' which may be required, including from experts.

Special 'preaction protocols' for personal injury and clinical negligence claims now form part of the rules of court: the protocols set out steps which should be followed before the claimant starts proceedings. For instance;

- the potential claimant should give the potential defendant three months to reply to "the letter of claim"

- if the defendant does not accept responsibility he should enclose with his reply to the letter of claim copies of the relevant documents concerning the accident/incident in his possession

- the parties should, especially in lower value claims likely to be allocated by the court to the Fast Track, try to agree to obtain only one medical and/or other expert report rather than each side obtaining their own expert's report – as this inevitably adds to the expense of the case.

If the steps in the protocols are not followed, the court has the power, if and when proceedings are started, to 'penalise' the 'guilty' party usually by requiring him to pay some of the other party's legal costs e.g for the extra work involved in obtaining two medical reports rather than one.

But whether a healthcare practitioner is asked to advise or prepare a report for both parties or only for one side, his role as an expert is to exercise clear professional and independent judgement. The party or parties and their solicitors need to know the weaknesses as well as the strengths of the case so that they can decide in a balanced way whether or how to proceed with the claim or defence, including whether to try and settle their differences.

The Civil Procedure Rules (Part 35) emphasise that once proceedings are started an expert witness' duty is to help the court and not primarily to work for or with whichever party sends him instructions or pays him.

Healthcare practitioners need to bear this in mind from the time they are first asked to advise on a potential case.

The other very important matter which each party and their solicitor will need to sort out at an early stage is how the cost of the legal work is to be paid for. Not many individuals can afford to fund a legal claim through to trial, particularly one that is strongly contested or is complicated. Only those who are not earning are financially eligible for Legal Aid*

From 2000 Legal Aid will not be available for most personal injury claims (one exception will be medical negligence claims). Potential claimants in accident cases may receive help from their trade union, some will have legal expenses insurance (as part of their house contents or car insurance) and many law firms now offer "no win – no fee" arrangements, often linked to special "after-the-event" legal expenses insurance, which will pay for items such as experts' fees, and cover the other party's costs if the claimant loses the case.

Most defendants to personal injury and clinical negligence claims will have insurance and the insurance company will decide whether to settle or defend the claim, and how it is to be run: they will appoint solicitors for the legal work.

Pre-action Disclosure of documents and inspection of property

If one party, often the claimant, wants to see papers (documents) which the other party has before starting a claim and the second party refuses to make them available (whether under the protocol procedure or otherwise) the first party can apply to the court for an order for the release of the documents, provided he/she can show it is really necessary to see the papers to settle or pursue the claim. The same principles/court rules apply if it is necessary for e.g factory machinery to be inspected/preserved as it was at the time of the accident.

Healthcare practitioners advising/preparing reports invariably need to see the claimant's medical records. These can usually be obtained by the claimant as of right (under the Data Protection Act 1998) but occasionally applications to court may be necessary if a healthcare body is slow in locating or providing the records or if a potential claimant does not provide the potential defendant with all the records he/she thinks are necessary

Issue of Proceedings

In both the County and High Court the issue of proceedings involves the solicitor taking or sending a claim form and a fee to the Court. The court will enter an action number on the form after sealing it with the court seal.

The claim form must contain:

- a concise statement of the nature of the claim and the remedy sought

- a statement of the likely value of the claim (to enable the court to allocate the case to a 'track' if it is defended)

- a 'statement of truth' i.e a statement that the claimant believes the facts stated are true

Full particulars of the claim may either be included on the claim form or sent to the court/the defendant within 14 days. The particulars are the claimants "statement of case" and should include

- his version of events

- specific allegations against the defendant

- reference to any applicable law

The particulars may also include or annex

- evidence e.g documents on which the claim is based

- witness statements

There are specific rules for some types of case e.g in a personal injury claim, a medical report and a schedule of losses must also be annexed to the particulars.

Under the CPR it is the court which serves the claim/particulars on the defendant(s) unless the claimant receives permission to do so.

The Defence

The Defendant must respond to the particulars of the claim (not the claim form without particulars) within 14 days. He can choose to

- admit the claim in whole or in part, or admit liability but dispute the amount claimed

- defend and/or counterclaim

- acknowledge service – if he does this his full defence must follow within 14 days unless the claimant is willing to agree an extension of time, which without the court's express approval, cannot be any longer than 28 days.

The CPR specifically require defendants to answer all the claimant's allegations and with reasons. 'Holding' or 'bare denial' defences will be rejected by the court. In fact the court now has very wide powers to 'strike out' any statement of case, by claimant or defendant, which does not comply with the rules or does not disclose a real claim or defence.

Defences must also contain signed "statements of truth". In personal injury cases if the defendant disputes the medical report or schedule of loss he should say so, again giving reasons.

Case Management by the Court

The civil justice reforms place on the court a new duty to manage and control all cases in accordance with the "overriding objective" – a set of guiding principles set out in Rule 1, and specific case management powers summarised in Rules 3 and 26, and with regard to the separate tracks (see above) in Rules 27–29. These important changes are designed to ensure cases no longer 'drift' or take years to reach a conclusion, and to prevent the work and legal costs becoming 'disproportionate' to the amount in dispute.

The Court's new powers include:

- ordering a 'stay' of the proceedings to allow parties to negotiate or mediate – initally for up to one month

- working with the parties to 'narrow' the issues in dispute

- taking decisions on paper applications only or holding hearings by telephone or video to save time and costs

- taking steps to balance the power and/or resources between the parties

- imposing penalties (sanctions) on a party for disregarding the rules or the court's orders and directions, which might be the payment of the costs of a step or stage regardless of who 'wins' the case, or an order preventing the party relying on evidence served late

- controlling the costs by setting 'budgets' or limiting the amount that can be recovered from the other side e.g in expert's fees

- doing anything else to progress the claim of its own initiative

A judge will look at each defended case and the allocation questionnaires filled in by both parties (see above) and will as a minimum do the following:

- allocate the case to one of the three tracks (see above)

- set a trial date, or at least a trial 'window' (a period of a few weeks within which the trial will take place). In Small Claims and Fast Track cases this will only be about 30 weeks ahead; a much tighter timetable than most litigants and solicitors are used to

- give directions for the conduct of the case until trial, including a timetable for serving the evidence – documents, witness statements, expert's reports etc

In more complex cases on the Multi Track or where there appear to be problems e.g where one or more parties has already spent a considerable amount in legal costs in comparison with the value of the claim, the judge will call a "case management conference" and may require the parties to attend as well as their lawyers. The judge will use the conference to try to narrow the issues in dispute, encourage the parties to settle, and to plan/direct the conduct of the case in a "proportionate" way. For instance the judge might decide that:

• the entire case could be determined by "summary judgement" where either the claim or defence appears to have little reasonable prospect of success

• a specific issue, or liability as a whole should be tried first, leaving the amount of damages if any to be resolved later.

Disclosure of documents

One of the directions which the court may give at an early stage will concern disclosure of documents. Where a pre-action protocol has been followed or the parties have already co-operated on the key information in the case, no more disclosure may be needed. In most cases, especially those on the Fast Track, the court will order "standard disclosure" of the documents on which each party is relying and those which adversely affect his case, or support the other party's case. Each party has a duty to search for the appropriate documents and has to provide a signed, certified "disclosure statement" with their list of documents.

This "standard disclosure" test is much narrower than the test which applied before the CPR came into force, which required all documents relevant to any issue in the case or which might establish a train of enquiry to be disclosed. Sometimes this lead to huge quantities of paperwork being provided, including to the court at trial, which did not really progress the case at all and increased delay and costs. The aim of the new rules is to cut down the paperwork to the essential.

But if "standard disclosure" does not provide some of the apparently necessary information, or one party is concerned that the other has not 'searched' sufficiently thoroughly the court can order additional 'specific disclosure' or a 'further search' provided the amount in dispute and the work involved justify this.

Sometimes expert witnesses may need to advise a party about the documents which the other party should have and should disclose. Frequently the expert witness will need to see some of both parties' disclosure documents before finalising his report.

Not all documents concerning a case have to be subject to the disclosure test – in particular letters between the solicitor and the client once proceedings are planned or are highly likely, and sometimes letters to others, or a report providing advice on future litigation, are "privileged": the reason for this is to encourage clients to tell their legal advisors the full truth, and to enable the lawyers to advise the clients as frankly as possible, particularly about the weaknesses of the case. Drafts of witness statements or expert's reports are not usually required to be disclosed either. An expert witness should check with the solicitor if in doubt about whether documents sent to him should be referred to in a report – because once referred to "privilege" attaching to the document may be 'waived'.

Settlement

The vast majority of civil cases settle before trial (and many before the action has started). This means the parties come to an agreement to end the legal proceedings. It is in the interests of both parties to reach a settlement rather than to have to spend time and money on a trial.

There are many opportunities to reach a settlement as the litigation progresses and the CPR expressly encourage this. It is often possible to settle cases after disclosure of some or all of the evidence. Each side can assess the relative strength and weaknesses of his case. The expert's role in reaching settlement can be crucial. An expert's report that identifies all the strengths of the case and is able to deal effectively with any areas of weakness is an essential tool in reaching settlement.

Under the previous rules of court defendants could try to settle a claim by paying into court the amount of money which they thought the claim was worth or which the claimant might accept. If the claimant accepted the money and the parties sorted out who paid the legal costs the case would end, usually with a "consent order" which the court would endorse.

If the claimant did not accept the money and the case continued to trial:

- if the judge awarded the claimant more than the amount in court the claimant would also receive (nearly) all his costs from the defendant

- but if the judge awarded less than the amount in court, the claimant would usually have to pay the defendant's costs from the date when the money was paid in, and would not receive any contribution to his own costs from that date either

The judge would not be told about the amount in court until after the trial when he would make the decisions about the costs.

Although this system provided a powerful incentive to defendants to try to settle claims, it did not give claimants any opportunity to put similar pressure on defendants. So an important innovation in Part 360 of the CPR is the "claimants' offer to settle" – a claimant can now, at any time, even before starting proceedings, make the defendant an offer. If this is not accepted and the case goes to trial the judge, as with a payment in, will not be told of the offer and

- if the judge awards the claimant as much or more than their own offer, the defendant will usually be ordered to pay additional money to the claimant – up to an extra 10% interest on the damages, and all the claimant's costs, plus additional interest on those as well

The new rules also permit defendants to make offers to settle, including pre-action, but to be effective they should be followed up by a payment into court when proceedings have been started.

The new offer to settle rules should lead to many more cases settling and at an earlier stage, thus reducing delay and saving costs and leading to happier clients.

The court also has new powers in the CPR to specifically encourage settlements, especially by ordering a 'stay of proceedings' to enable parties to hold a negotiation meeting or mediation, or use another form of alternative dispute resolution (see below). This approach has been adopted in the Commercial Court for some time and has worked very well – with a high percentage of cases settling before trial.

'Without prejudice' documents produced with a view to settlement are protected by privilege (see above). In the event of negotiations being unsuccessful these documents cannot be referred to at trial but can be when it comes to settling the costs of the case.

The later stages of an action

If a case has not settled after the evidence has been exchanged, the court will send the parties a "listing questionnaire" to complete about 8 – 10 weeks before the trial date. This will act as a check on whether the previous directions have all been compiled with, and will be the parties final opportunity to seek further directions particularly concerning who will attend and give oral evidence at the trial, including expert witnesses. The court will then fix a definite trial date (if this has not been done before).

In more complex cases a further "case management conference" called a pre-trial review (PTR) may be arranged to plan the trial itself – the judge may require the parties to produce for the PTR or at trial

- a chronology of events

- a short statement of the remaining disputed issues

- "skeleton arguments" i.e a note summarising the arguments to be put orally by the advocates

- details of any case authorities to be relied upon

- a 'reading plan' to enable the trial judge to read the key documents before the trial

A civil trial

Usually the claimant's advocate makes an opening speech. He or she explains the facts to the judge and sets out the issues in dispute. The defence may make an opening speech but not as a matter of routine.

The next stage is that the claimant's witnesses give evidence. Each witness may be examined-in-chief by the claimant's lawyer and then cross-examined by the defendant's lawyer. (The witness may be re-examined by the claimant's lawyer if anything new has come up in the cross-examination that requires clarification).

Then the defendant's witnesses give evidence, in the same way.

Finally, there will be closing speeches. The defendant's advocate usually speaks first and is followed by the claimant's advocate.

It is important to note that disclosure of documents, the exchange of witness of fact statements, expert reports and if ordered 'skeleton arguments' means that each party should know in advance what oral evidence the witnesses will give. In addition, the judge will take into account the evidence given in the witness box when reaching his decision.

Evidence in civil trials

Evidence in civil trials can be divided into three categories:

• Witness evidence

• Documents

• Real evidence

A witness of fact is someone who is called to give evidence in a case about what happened. They are there to recall what they saw or heard. They are not generally allowed to give opinion evidence. This should be contrasted with an expert witness who may give both factual and opinion evidence.

Two examples of witnesses of fact in civil cases are the witness who sees a car accident in which the claimant is injured and the witness who recalls the medical advice given to a patient who is claiming for professional negligence.

A witness of fact will frequently give oral evidence at trial. This is because oral evidence is deemed to be the best form of evidence as it can be tested under cross-examination. The witness who gives oral evidence in the witness box may refresh his memory from any contemporaneous notes he has kept.

Contemporaneous records are records completed while the facts were still fresh in the witness's mind. Such a contemporaneous note is part of the oral evidence and may be read out by the witness. The other party has the right to request and inspect such contemporaneous notes. Examples of such notes are medical records.

Where an expert is to give factual evidence it is important for him or her to keep accurate and full notes. The following information is important.

- Dates, times, locations

- Who was present (e.g. other staff)

- Inspections

- Details of observed facts and, if an expert, his/her opinion on the facts

- Detail of conversations / advice given

Witness statements

A witness statement by witnesses of fact is made. It will usually be written some time after the events it records, once litigation seems likely or has begun. The purpose of a witness statement is to set out in writing the details of a particular event or series or events of which the witness has first hand knowledge.

Under the CPR the court controls the numbers of witnesses of fact from whom witness statements are required or who may be allowed to give oral evidence at the trial. The parties are required to put their proposals to the court in the allocation questionnaire and the court then gives directions. Usually the court will order "witness statements" to be exchanged within a few weeks of any disclosure of documents. The rules set out specific requirements for the format and content of witness statements – in particular they should be as concise as possible and in the witnesses own words and must conclude with a "statement of truth".

Increasingly to save time at the trial a witness statement will 'stand as evidence' and will take the place of examination-in-chief (questions asked by the lawyer of the party who calls the witness).

Further, if the statement is not controversial and the other side does not wish to cross-examine the witness about it, the statement may be included in the trial papers without the necessity of the witness attending. A witness statement is always available for the witness to refresh his memory from before he goes into the witness box to give evidence.

Expert evidence

An expert witness may give evidence of both fact and opinion. The expert must take great care to identify the source of the facts on which he or she bases the expert opinion. Facts, which the expert has observed first hand, will usually be given greater weight than facts that the expert has been told by another person. The reliability of information reported to an expert by another person may be tested at trial by the cross-examination of the person who supplied this information to the expert.

Expert opinion evidence may be admissible on matters not within the common knowledge of the court. It can be based upon experiment, experience, research or the work of others. The expert is entitled to give such opinion evidence because of his qualifications and experience in his field of expertise.

Lord Woolf, during his "Access to Justice" enquiry, became particularly concerned that too frequently parties in civil claims introduced expert evidence which was not necessary, and which sometimes was 'tailored' to meet the party's case rather than give an independent unbiased opinion. He concluded that the over-adversarial use of expert evidence, and on occasions over-adversarial conduct of experts themselves, was a factor in the delays and high cost of some litigation.

Accordingly the CPR gives the case managing judge very specific powers to control which expert evidence can be introduced, both in terms of numbers and types of expert, and the costs of this which may be recovered from the losing party.

The rules also stress that an expert's duty is to assist the court, not the party who instructs or pays him, and set out very specific requirements for the content and format of an expert's report including that:

- it must contain a summary of the material instructions, on the basis of which the report was written

- the expert should set out the range of professional opinion on important issues, stating where his own opinion lies within that range, with reasons

- it must conclude with both a declaration that the expert understands his duty to the court and a statement of truth

The rules also require parties to try, whenever possible, to 'share' expert evidence by jointly instructing a single expert from a particular discipline, rather than one each. The court has the express power to order that expert evidence will only be admissible from a single expert. This will be the usual order in the Fast Track, where oral evidence from an expert at trial will also be the exception. In larger more complex cases the court may nonetheless order that only one report from a single expert will be allowed on technical or valuation issues.

Other ways in which the court will seek to economise on expert evidence and/or encourage experts on opposing sides to reach agreement will include:

- one party disclosing their expert's reports before the other – the second party might decide he/she does not need an expert at all

- both parties asking written questions of the experts on their reports to a tight timetable

SBRLSMD (Whitechapel)

Civil litigation: overview of the basic procedure

Information collected (possibly including an expert's preliminary report)

↓

Protocol followed or
Letter of claim + response

↓

Negotiations/attempt to settle

↓

Issue and service of claim and particulars
(with the expert's medical report and schedule of damages)

↓

Defence (and counterclaim)

↓

Allocation to track, (+case management conference),
directions + trial window/date fixed

↓

Disclosure + service of witness statements and expert reports which are going
to be relied on at the trial

↓

Return of listing questionnaires, (PTR) + trial date confirmed
Prepare for trial [often settlement]

↓

Trial

- ordering the experts to hold a discussion/meeting before the trial to try to narrow down the areas of disagreement. The outcome will not bind the parties but a note of the meeting will have to be produced and kept on the court file

- placing a limit on the amount of expert's fees which may be recoverable from the other party even if the case is won

Other types of evidence used in civil trials

Documentary evidence

This includes photographs, video recordings and tape recordings as well as paper documents (e.g. letters, internal memoranda, hospital notes) made by the parties themselves during the period which is the focus of the action. The court may make an order that a particular document be disclosed.

What is legal aid?

Where a person cannot afford the full legal fees involved in litigation, he may apply for legal aid. This is taxpayers' money and is distributed by the Legal Aid Board. A solicitor will apply to the Legal Aid Board for legal aid, giving details of the case. The Legal Aid Board will analyse the application and decide whether it is in the interests of justice that taxpayers' money should be used to fund litigation and also whether the applicant could pay something towards those legal costs. The costs of experts' reports may be covered by Legal Aid. The solicitor can get 'prior approval' from the Legal Aid Board and experts should insist on this being done to ensure they are paid. If there is no prior approval, the Board may disallow the expert's fees and he or she will then have to claim the fee from the solicitor.

What is alternative dispute resolution (ADR)?

Because of the cost of legal proceedings, many civil cases are now being dealt with through means other than the traditional court system. These include mediation and other means of A.D.R. such as expert determination or early neutral evaluation.

The purpose of A.D.R. is to enable parties to settle their disputes by using a third party to act as a mediator, arbitrator or evaluator. The mediator does not give a binding judgement but assists the parties to reach a settlement. The parties can proceed to or with the litigation if they are unable to reach agreement. The advantage of A.D.R. is that it is quicker, cheaper and less formal than court proceedings. It is particularly suitable for parties who wish to retain a working relationship after the dispute is over. Sometimes a contract between two parties will provide for A.D.R. in the event of a contractual dispute. Alternatively, the parties can simply agree to use A.D.R. instead of or during litigation through the court system.

Mediation

Mediation is probably the best known and most widely used of a number of alternative dispute resolution procedures. It is a process in which disputing parties meet privately before an independent neutral, the mediator, to discuss their differences and seek a solution with her assistance. It should be stressed that the essence of mediation is that the mediator is not a judge or arbitrator. She does not determine the issues, but facilitates a solution arrived at voluntarily by the parties. The English courts may order the parties to a dispute to refer their case to a mediator to seek a settlement before the court hears the case. Mediation is a flexible, economic and confidential approach which allows the parties to retain control of the matter until they reach agreement. In England and Wales the premier independent bodies supporting and promoting alternative dispute resolution are the Centre For Dispute Resolution (CEDR), a registered charity solicitor which provide mediation information and services, and the ADR Group, a network of solicitor mediators. Both bodies train and accredit mediators. Experts are not usually required to attend a mediation.

Arbitration

In contrast to mediation, the results of an arbitration are binding. An arbitrator is chosen by the parties in dispute to settle their differences. Experts may be involved in giving evidence and the procedures are in many respects similar to traditional court proceedings. Often the arbitrator is himself a specialist on the matters in dispute which means that the expert does not have to explain the technical matters that a non-expert would need to know.

What is the procedure in criminal cases?

Magistrates Court

All criminal cases start with initial proceedings in the Magistrates Court. The Magistrates will decide whether a defendant is to be held in custody to await trial or whether the defendant will be granted bail. They also decide if a defendant is entitled to legal aid. Finally they have to decide whether the defendant's trial will take place in the Magistrates Court or in the Crown Court.

Criminal trials that take place in the Magistrates Court are called summary trials. They concern the less serious sorts of crimes. There will usually be three lay magistrates. These will be three non-lawyers who have volunteered to sit as Justices of the Peace. They will be assisted in matters of law and practice by a legally qualified Magistrates Clerk. Sometimes, instead of three lay magistrates there will be one stipendiary magistrate sitting alone. He or she will be a qualified barrister or solicitor with at least 7 years experience. They should be addressed as '*Sir*' or '*Madam*' but <u>not</u> as '*Your Worship.*'

The trial will be heard by the Magistrates and they will decide if the defendant is guilty or not guilty. The Magistrates will also pass sentence. They will often adjourn to get pre-sentence reports before passing sentence.

The Crown Court

The Crown Court tries the more serious crimes. Trial in the Crown Court is known as trial on indictment.

Who sits

There will be a judge (who may be a High Court judge, a circuit judge or a recorder). The judge directs the jury on the law and the weight of the evidence. The jury decides whether the defendant is guilty or not guilty. If the defendant is convicted, the judge passes sentence, usually after an adjournment for pre-sentence reports.

Correct form of address

This will depend on the status of the judge. Ask the usher or the lawyers. All judges sitting in the Crown Court (circuit judges, recorders and assistant recorders) are addressed as '*Your honour*' except High Court (or red) judges and any judge sitting at the Old Bailey in London or in the court of the Recorder of Liverpool or Manchester. These judges are all addressed as '*Your lordship/ladyship.*' A High Court judge is often referred to as a 'red judge' because his formal court attire is coloured red (and black). On the court list, a High Court judge's surname is always followed by the abbreviation 'J.', as opposed to the abbreviation 'H.H.J.' used for circuit judges.

The High Court

Appeals from the Magistrates Court or the Crown Court may sometimes be heard in the Queen's Bench Division of the High Court.

Who sits

One High Court judge and one Lord Justice of Appeal.

Correct form of address

'*Your Lordship/Ladyship.*'

The Court of Appeal

The Criminal Division hears appeals from the Crown Court on points of law and also appeals against sentence by the prosecution or the defence.

Who sits

Usually three but sometimes two judges. At least one of these judges must be a Lord Justice of Appeal. The other judges may be either one circuit judge, up to two High Court Judges or up to two Lord Justices of Appeal. The Lord Chief Justice is a Lord Justice of Appeal. He is also the head of the Criminal Division of the Supreme Court, i.e., he is the most senior criminal judge in England and Wales.

Correct form of address

'Your Lordship/Ladyship.'

The House of Lords

Like the Court of Appeal, the House of Lords is exclusively appellate. It hears appeals from the Court of Appeal (Criminal Division) and also (exceptionally) from the Queen's Bench Division of the High Court.

Who sits

Three to seven, but usually five Lords of Appeal.

Correct form of address

'Your Lordship/Ladyship.'

Parties to proceedings in the Criminal Courts

The Prosecution

The Crown Prosecution Service prosecutes people for allegedly committing crimes. At the trial, the prosecution's case is heard first. There are other prosecuting authorities.

The Defendant

The defendant in a criminal trial is a person whom the prosecution alleges has committed a criminal offence. Criminal offences are set out in statutes (i.e. Acts of Parliament) or exist as common-law offences; that is, they are offences that have been created by the judges in decided cases. The defendant may be found 'guilty' or 'not guilty'. This is a decision made by the jury in the Crown Court and by the Magistrates in the Magistrates Court. Once a defendant has been found guilty, there will be a further hearing in court to decide on the sentence. Sentences may be custodial or non-custodial; that is the defendant can be imprisoned or can receive a sentence falling short of imprisonment, (e.g. a fine or a community sentence).

The burden and standard of proof

Generally the burden (or onus) of proof rests on the prosecution. The prosecution is required to prove every fact in issue to a high standard, (i.e. beyond a reasonable doubt) in order to secure a conviction. This burden extends not only to proving every element of the offence, but also to disproving the defendant's defence.

Where the prosecution must prove their case beyond a reasonable doubt the jury or magistrates should convict only if they are sure that the defendant is guilty. By contrast, where the defence is required to prove its defence on the balance of probability, the jury or magistrates should accept this defence only if they are satisfied that the defence is more likely to be true than not.

How do Criminal Cases Start?

Criminal cases generally start with investigations by the police. If, after investigation, it is believed that an individual has committed an offence, then that individual will either be sent a summons (this is usual in less serious offences such as careless driving), or the individual will be arrested and then (usually after a police interview) charged with an offence or released.

The initial proceeding for all cases will take place in the Magistrates Court. The magistrates will decide if the defendant is entitled to be released on bail pending trial, or whether the defendant will be held in custody to await trial. The magistrates will also decide if the defendant is entitled to have Criminal Legal Aid to defend the case. This decision will be based partly on the means of the defendant and partly on whether it is in the 'interests of justice' that the defendant should receive Legal Aid.

For summary only offences and 'either way' offences not committed to the Crown Court, the summary trial takes place in the Magistrates Court. From the Magistrates Court or the Crown Court there may be appeals to the higher courts.

What is the role of a healthcare practitioner who acts as an expert witness?

Definition of an expert witness

Expert witnesses are individuals with qualifications and experience that enable them to give an opinion on the facts of a case. They are only entitled to give evidence on a particular specialist field which will be defined by their qualifications and experience. Firstly, it is their role to help the party and lawyers understand technical matters. Secondly, they may advise on the strength and weaknesses of the case. They may also assist lawyers in the drafting of legal documents such as statements of case. They produce evidence in two forms:

- the written report (or occasionally a witness statement)
- oral evidence at a court hearing or trial.

As well as appropriate qualifications and experience in their own professional field, they may also be members of an expert witness organisation.

Many cases raise healthcare issues. This is where the expert can play a vital part. His or her prime role is to identify, simplify and explain these matters for the court. Many lay people, lawyers, and even judges will not understand the matters without the assistance of the expert.

It is the duty of all expert witnesses to help the court on the matters relevant to their specific areas of expertise. The expert should be impartial, independent and truthful. This duty over-rides any obligation to the person from whom he or she has received instructions.

Courts will restrict expert evidence to that which is reasonably required to resolve the proceedings justly. The courts are concerned to keep costs of litigation to the absolute minimum. Experts' fees can be substantial. No party can put in an expert's report as evidence without the court's permission.

The expert should give the instructing lawyer an unbiased opinion. In order to make sure that experts are independent, courts would prefer the use of experts to be as transparent as possible. The following quote from The Ikarian Reefer 1993 (2) Lloyds Reports 68 is relevant:

> *'It is necessary that expert evidence presented to the court should be and should be seen to be the independent product of the expert uninfluenced as to form or content via the exigencies of litigation.'*

The initial instructions

Generally, the first contact between the expert and the instructing solicitor will be a telephone call. The instructing solicitor will wish to confirm the expert's suitability for the case, and availability to prepare a report within the required timescale and the appropriateness of his or her expertise. Further, he will wish to ensure that the expert does not have any conflicts of interest.

The instructions will then be confirmed in a letter of instruction from the solicitor to the expert.

Conflicts of interest

As noted, the expert should assist the court impartially. He or she must therefore be (and be perceived to be) independent. For this reason, before accepting appointment, an expert should ensure that there are no conflicts of interest. If there are, he or she should decline to act. An example might be working for the health trust that is involved in the litigation. However, in certain cases after full disclosure of the conflict to the instructing solicitors, he or she may act.

2

Organising an expert witness practice

Aims

This chapter will help you to

- Understand the organisational requirements of an expert witness practice

- Decide the personnel needed to run a practice

- Decide what reference material you need to have

- Decide the need for, and use of, information technology.

Why do you need to be organised ?

Most healthcare professionals begin as expert witnesses in a haphazard manner with the occasional request for a report or opinion.

Some never wish for more and, for them, the need for organisation around all other professional and personal activities is simple. They need only make time available when necessary.

However, if the healthcare professional wishes to have an expert witness practice, it is essential to undertake the organisation of the practice as early as possible.

Without an organised practice, neither the healthcare professional nor the solicitors who instruct them will be able to function to the best of their ability; important deadlines will be missed and the healthcare professional may find the supply of instructions dries up as their disorganisation becomes known among solicitors and to the courts.

What elements need to be organised?

In order to manage an expert witness practice which functions efficiently, allowing time for other professional and personal activity, the following broad areas need to be organised

- Time
- Facilities
- Secretarial support
- Technological aids
- Financial management

Time management

There are only 168 hours in the week and the healthcare professional must not only fit in all professional and personal activities but they must also find time for the expert witness practice.

When you begin there may be so little work that it can be handled in a haphazard way. However, as the workload increases, it will either impose on your professional or your free and personal time if you fail to get organised.

Most healthcare professionals do not give up their vocation to become expert witnesses full-time and indeed, to maintain credibility, most solicitors will only use professionals who have an active clinical practice. Therefore, time either has to be made available during the working day (by reducing or reorganising one's professional life) while still complying with the contract of employment or this work must be done outside those contracted hours. If a regular number of hours can be set aside for such work with the knowledge and recognition of your employers then the amount of work achieved will probably be greater than if the same amount of time was fitted in around all other activities in the working week.

Facilities required for an expert practice

One priority for an expert witness practice is to enable easy contact by solicitors. Therefore a healthcare professional setting out needs a contact address and facilities where he/she can be reached on a regular basis.

The choice of the contact address is important. If the healthcare professional is in private practice then all expert witness work will be addressed through these premises. If, however, they are employed within an organisation and do not have their own office, then the use of the hospital address for correspondence can cause problems.

If the practice also uses the facilities of a private hospital or consulting rooms, this would be the appropriate address. Otherwise, it may be appropriate for some individuals to use their home address.

Having established a contact address, the next priority is a method of oral communication and contact, particularly when urgent. Again, a contact phone number either manned or using an answering machine that can be accessed from a remote phone at regular intervals is important. If an answering service or secretary is used as the contact point, then they should always know how to contact the healthcare professional urgently. Email will soon be essential.

While the facilities of a personal mobile phone may suit some people as a contact point, this can be intrusive and may lead to resentment or, in some hospital environments, even interfere with electrical equipment. It may not, therefore, be a foolproof method of contact.

The third aspect is a place to see patients, if and when appropriate, and to write reports. Again, both of these may be done in an office at the place of employment (assuming that this is allowed within your contract and any fees due for the use of the facilities are met) or a room made available at home and used as an office.

Another option is to book a room either on an *ad hoc* or regular basis within a private hospital or consulting rooms.

Secretarial support

While the occasional request for an expert report may be met by the *ad hoc* use of your own secretary, their first priority is to their employer, and any other work must be done outside their working hours. With a computer, the fledgling expert may feel able to undertake most of the secretarial work themselves. As the work increases, however, the other administrative tasks (e.g. making appointments, answering requests, looking for medical records and keeping deadlines) will also increase. This may soon overwhelm the expert working alone and some support will be necessary.

The advantage of using a secretary exclusively for expert witness work is that they develop a loyalty to that work and are able to give it their whole attention. It also means that no conflict of interest arises between the normal employment and the expert witness work. The disadvantages of employing a secretary is the cost and that they will require to a place to work.

Do I need a computer ?

Many healthcare professionals now have access to a computer for their normal daily work and may even have one at home.

While the production of high quality reports is possible without such technology, the many revisions necessary while preparing such a report are made much easier with a computer. There are standard report formats (see **Appendix A**) which will speed up the writing of reports. These are also sold in disc form (See Appendix D).

The CPR Practice Direction on Expert Evidence also sets out specific requirements for reports prepared for use in court.

The production of any standard letters (replying to letters of instruction and giving appointments) are less time-consuming with a computer.

A dictation machine will be necessary if one uses a secretary as will the transcription machine for the secretary to use. Voice recognition systems which allow direct dictation into the computer either for transcription later or correction while dictation are improving but are not, as yet, universally acknowledged as a useful tool.

Case management systems now being installed in lawyer's offices can be modified for use by an expert witness but this will only benefit the expert who has a steady supply of work.

How should I organise the finances of my practice ?

Getting paid for work in the legal field is an important subject and will be dealt with in greater detail later (see Chapter 13). However, it is appropriate to touch briefly on the organisational aspects of finances.

Unless the expert witness work is minimal, a separate bank account for all transactions related to this work should be opened. All income from this work should be paid into, and all expenses related to it should be taken out of this account.

As the new system of self-assessment is underway in

the UK there is a duty to keep records of all financial transactions and this applies to the management of an expert witness practice.

While a manual account book can be used and invoices prepared, a dedicated computer accounting package results in smoother management of the financial aspects and gives financial information to the healthcare professional about the practice at regular intervals, without the need for laborious manual calculations. Examples of these are Microsoft Money, Quickbooks (Intuit) and Mind Your Own Business (Apple Macintosh).

3

The coroner system

Aims

This chapter will help you

- To understand the differences between the coroner system and other legal fora

- To understand the role and limits of the coroners duties in relationship to healthcare professionals

- To prepare written and oral evidence to assist the coroner

Introduction

The coroner system is inquisitorial rather than adversarial system.

For the healthcare professional, however, there are pitfalls simply because of the nature of the proceedings.

While in other legal fora there are only two sides, in the coroners court, each of the parties with a legitimate interest can ask questions and be legally represented.

The coroner has great autonomy in his own court and the proceedings are controlled by him. The coroner is answerable to the Lord Chancellor and his decisions can be scrutinised by the High Court.

Preparing written evidence for the coroner.

The duty of the coroner is to investigate sudden, unexpected death. Many deaths reported to the coroner will have had a post mortem which shows the cause of death as natural. The coroner will be satisfied, and will allow a death certificate to be issued.

However, in certain deaths where there is concern, the coroner will institute enquiries and will begin by asking the healthcare professionals involved with the person's care prior to death for a written statement. In some cases, the coroner may also ask more senior professionals not directly involved in the person's care but responsible for policy making in a healthcare facility, for statements. These statements may be about the care given and/or the policies in force with regard to specific aspects of that care.

In most cases, a factual statement similar to a police statement, is all that may be required and the same format as the section 9 declaration will be sufficient (**Figure 3.1**).

The statement should include who you are, including any professional qualifications and the position you hold. You should then inform the coroner when and how you were involved with the deceased person and what care you rendered to them.

> I am Joan Jones, a registered general nurse, at present working on the acute admissions ward at St Elsewhere's Hospital Trust.
>
> On 27 December 1997 a patient known to us as Mr Symonds, DOB 10/01/20 was admitted directly to the ward having been found at home unconscious. On initial assessment his clothes were ragged and his rectal temperature was 34 C.
>
> He was in an unkempt state and there were multiple abrasions and bruises of differing colours noted when he was undressed. He was covered in excrement and his clothes smelt of urine.
>
> Despite measures to rewarm him over the next 24 hours and full supportive measures he did not regain consciousness and died on the 28th December. He was taken from the ward to the mortuary having been laid out by myself and a colleague.

Figure 3.1 Example statement

If the healthcare professional suspects that there may be accusations of inadequate treatment, this statement should be written after taking legal advice. The advice should be taken from a representative of the Defence Society, a professional organisation or the legal department of your employers. It should be noted, however, that in a potential conflict of interest between your employers and the individual healthcare professional, the hospital trust may decline to provide legal support, either for the preliminary stages or to represent the healthcare professional at the inquest. If the individual does not have a professional indemnity insurance, the cost of privately financing representation may be prohibitive.

After assessing all statements, the coroner may convene an inquest.

Appearing at an inquest

The coroner will convene an inquest if he has doubts as to the cause of death or if there is a legitimate public interest in the cause of death. Should criminal proceedings be pending, the inquest will be formally opened and then adjourned to allow the deceased to be released to relatives for burial.

This is because while the coroner is investigating the cause of death he is not establishing blame in a criminal sense for the death. Therefore certain verdicts which the coroner could give for a death could influence the outcome of criminal proceedings if the inquest preceded a criminal trial.

An inquest may be held with the coroner acting alone or with a jury of between 7 and 11 people.

While some major cities have coroner's courts, many inquests are held in the building where the coroner practices or in a solicitor's practice. Wherever the court is sitting, it is nevertheless a court with all the usual judicial sanctions.

The coroner may call witnesses or, alternatively, read statements previously submitted.

Any witnesses called by the coroner will be sent a witness summons (**Figure 3.2**).

If there is any doubt as to the cause of death or there may be some liability in the death by an individual, it may be wise to have legal representation at the inquest. This may be provided by the legal representatives of your employer or, if your own actions are being examined, it may be provided by your professional indemnity scheme.

Preparing for the inquest.

Before the inquest, ensure that you have any clinical records for the patient and any statements that have been prepared by members of the hospital staff not being called to the inquest.

If you are being represented at the inquest, it is worthwhile having a meeting with your legal representative. Identify any potential problems in your evidence and prepare questions for any other parties present at the inquest.

Attending the inquest

On the day of the inquest, arrive in good time for the start of the proceedings and find your legal representative.

St. Elsewhere Metropolitan Borough Council

Coroner's District – St. Elsewhere South

Witness Summons

To ....

of

....

YOU ARE HEREBY SUMMONED to appear before me on

the .... day of .... 19....... at ....
am/pm

at the Council Chamber, St. Elsewhere Council House, High Street, St. Elsewhere, to give

evidence touching the death of

DATED this .... day of .... 19........

H.M.Coroner

St Elsewhere (South)

(Note: Failure to comply with this summons may render the person liable to a fine not exceeding £400) (Coroners Act 1887 s.19)

....

PLEASE SIGN THIS PORTION AND RETURN TO THE CORONER'S OFFICE IN THE ENVELOPE PROVIDED NO LATER THAN FIVE DAYS AFTER RECEIPT.

H M Coroners Officer

St Elsewhere Police Station

St Elsewhere

Sir,

I acknowledge receipt of a summons to attend H M Coroners Court being held at

(time) .... on (date) ....

at (place) ....

Full Name..

Signature..

Date returned...

Figure 3.2 Sample witness summons

In the room where the inquest is to be held there may be a formal arrangement similar to a court or a more informal seating arrangement.

At most proceedings you will sit with your legal representative. If evidence is presented by anyone else during the inquest which you feel requires an explanation, your legal representative may ask questions and you can pass notes to your legal representative to help them with this questioning.

Presenting your evidence.

As in all courts, evidence is presented under oath and when asked to give evidence you will be asked to take the oath. This is slightly different from the oath taken in court (**Figure 3.3**). However, as the coroners court is a judicial body anyone giving knowingly untruthful evidence is liable for prosecution under the offence of perjury.

Initially the coroner will take you through your evidence. He may ask specific questions to clarify any points which appear unclear in the evidence. After the coroner has asked his questions, your legal representative, the legal representatives of any other parties present and any parties not legally represented can ask questions, if allowed to do so, by the coroner.

When all the evidence has been presented, the coroner will summarize the evidence and make a decision as to the cause of death.

There are a limited list of verdicts that the coroner can return (see opposite).

I swear by Almighty God that the evidence I shall give at this inquiry (inquest) shall be the truth the whole truth and nothing but the truth.

Figure 3.3 The oath in coroners court

List of possible verdicts following an inquest

Natural causes

Unlawful killing

Accident

Misadventure

Neglect

Killed him/her self

Industrial disease

Abuse of drugs

Want of attention at birth

Abortion

Jury inquest

If the coroner sits with a jury, the jury will decide the cause of death having been advised by the coroner on the possible verdicts they can return.

What can happen after an inquest ?

Following an inquest, various actions may occur. The coroner may make recommendations as to a suggested course of action that an authority may follow such as the road layout in the case of a fatal accident in a roadway or suggestions about the equipment on vehicles which have safety implications.

If there is evidence of lack of care to a specific nature or evidence of criminal wrongdoing, the coroner can refer his findings to the Crown Prosecution service for them to assess whether a criminal prosecution is needed. This could happen in the case of carbon monoxide poisoning in a rented property with regard to the landlord's responsibility.

If, during an inquest, there is evidence that negligence has occurred, including employer's liability, road traffic accidents where an individual can be responsible or deficiencies in the medical care of a patient prior to death, the next of kin may take legal advice in order to commence legal proceedings for damages either for personal injury or medical negligence.

It is therefore not unusual if there is a suspicion of someone at 'fault' for the death that the family has representation at the inquest from lawyers. These lawyers can often use the verdict of the inquest to aid them in the decision-making process regarding further civil proceedings.

Written evidence for criminal proceedings

Aims

This chapter will help you to

- Prepare written witness statements of fact for criminal proceedings

- Understand the rights of the police with regard to a patient undergoing medical treatment and the implications for a healthcare professional treating the patient

- Understand the reasons for the appointment of healthcare professionals as expert witnesses for the criminal courts

- Prepare expert reports for criminal proceedings.

Introduction

Who is responsible for prosecutions in England & Wales?

The prosecution of criminal offences is generally controlled by the Crown Prosecution Service (CPS), a body set up by an act of Parliament in 1985 which became fully operational in 1986. They receive the evidence concerning crime and make the decision on whether or not to proceed with the case against an individual.

Who provides the evidence to the Crown Prosecution Service?

The police gather evidence to present to the CPS to enable them to decide on the charges. In the case of injuries, the police normally approach healthcare professionals to obtain statements detailing the injuries.

In these circumstances, the healthcare professional is providing clinical evidence regarding the injuries received by a client or information on specific aspects of the care the client was given.

While the victim of a crime may be able to describe the injuries they suffered, they are not in a position to fully know the extent of their injuries or, more specifically, the treatment required. For this reason, healthcare professionals have to describe the injuries and their treatment because this requires skills and knowledge which a lay person does not have.

The description of the injuries received and the necessary treatment given to the patient indicates the seriousness of the injuries. When this information is presented to the CPS it may influence the charge that a person faces and can therefore influence the sentence that they may receive if found guilty.

In these circumstances the healthcare professional is being a 'witness of fact'.

What is a 'witness of fact'?

A 'witness of fact' is someone called to give evidence in a case about what actually happened. They are there to recall what they saw, heard or did during an incident. A 'witness of fact' will be required to discuss facts only as remembered or recorded in their notes.

How are you asked to provide a statement?

For doctors, most requests for statements regarding patients who have been treated in hospital are co-ordinated through an administrative channel. The police will request a statement from the doctor(s) involved in the case.

In serious cases, particularly where evidence such as clothes, personal effects or samples are taken by the police, other healthcare professionals may be asked to give a statement outlining their involvement in the case. In these circumstances, the most important part of collecting the evidence linking a suspect to the crime may be the circumstances of that crime. It is important for the prosecuting authorities to show an uninterrupted and complete record of the movement of a piece of evidence including all of the individuals who touched it. This is needed to show whether evidence was tampered with or whether it has remained unchanged until a forensic scientist has had a chance to examine it.

Most statements are compiled from the clinical notes made on a patient. These notes should be made at the time of contact with the patient or written up shortly after contact. It is important that all clinical records are dated and signed by the person writing them. It may be difficult to remember when compiling notes, in the midst of trying to treat a patient, that the most important thing that may be asked in the future may appear clinically insignificant during that first examination.

With some serious offences, particularly murder, a statement may be requested shortly after the event, when the memory of it is still clear. However, it is not unusual for a statement request to be delayed by weeks or even months.

In such cases, the memory is likely to have faded and the only record of your involvement and findings are the written notes made at the time. This again emphasises the importance of good note-taking. If the contemporaneous notes are unclear, brief or if you are unable to remember the particular patient, do not be tempted to add anything that you cannot clearly remember. If you have any doubts, talk to someone more senior than yourself or ask advice from the legal advisor of your employer or professional indemnity insurer. You may want to attend training on Healthcare Records run through your hospital by Bond Solon Training (See Appendix D).

Medical evidence in most criminal cases is judged purely on the written evidence and the legal profession try not to involve healthcare professionals in the court hearing. However, if the statements give cause for concern, either from the prosecution or the defence, the writer may be required to appear in court. By that time the memory may have faded further.

What do I need to do before writing a statement?

Before preparing a statement, make sure that you have all of the relevant clinical records. Make sure that, as a 'witness of fact,' you were personally involved and able to clarify the position.

While some clinical records may be available, there may be specific problems in obtaining all of the notes. It is important that the statement you make is compiled from your own notes and if you are unable to give a complete history of the treatment (e.g. the patient was transferred to another team), do not add details to your statement that you cannot confirm in court.

Check for patient consent if you are disclosing clinical data from medical records. In most cases, the police obtain consent for release of medical evidence during a witness statement from the patient and this may be appended to the request. It is advisable to have written consent, and to keep this with the copy of the statement you retain, as this is a dispute which may end up in court. If there is no consent, telephone the police officer concerned and ask them to obtain it.

If the patient has subsequently died and consent cannot be obtained, there are some circumstances where clinical details may be divulged as a matter of public interest. However, it would be wise for the healthcare professional to discuss this, either with their professional organisation (e.g. The Medical Defence Union or Royal College of Nursing) or the statutory body regulating their practice (e.g. The General Dental Council) before releasing any information to the prosecuting authorities.

How do I prepare a statement?

While hand-written statements are acceptable it is better if these are typewritten as this prevents transcription errors later. Occasionally, the police ask for statements at the time and they will write the statement for you. If you wish to write the statement (which we would recommend) ask the police to return after you have had time for preparation.

In order to comply with court proceedings, most statements are written on standard paper. This includes a standard declaration known as a 'Section 9 declaration' (**Figure 4.1**) on the first page. This is part of the Criminal Justice Act, 1967 and statements in this form are acceptable to the court. These can be read out in court and have the same weight as if the person is

---

Witness Statement

(C.J. Act 1967, s9; M.C. Rules 1981, r.70)
(Magistrates Courts Act 1980 s102)

Statement of.. *Age*..................

This statement (consisting of ... pages each signed by me) is true to the best of my knowledge and belief and I make it knowing that, if it is tendered in evidence, I shall be liable to prosecution if I have wilfully stated in it anything which I know to be false or do not believe to be true.

Dated .... *Signed* ....

Figure 4.1 'Section 9 Declaration'

present giving oral evidence, provided both sides in the court agree to the contents of the statement.

What should the statement of a doctor contain?

The first part of the statement should show who you are and your qualifications (without abbreviations). This should include the position you hold with relevance to the reason for the report. Although not necessary, some indication of your experience, time since qualification, further examinations and any specialist knowledge you may have can aid the legal team when they come to assess the contents of the statement.

The statement should then identify the client by name and date of birth (not address). You should note the date, place and time you examined the patient, if the records are available, and record these details (**Figure 4.2**).

Many notes, particularly relating to the emergency treatment, do not include all of these details and sometimes the exact timing of events may be important in the case. If they are not included in the medical statements, the practitioner may be called to court.

You should then record the patient complaint and why they presented. This is, of course, something that you cannot know first-hand as you were not present at the incident. As such it is hearsay (you have heard this story from another individual, not witnessed it yourself). You cannot therefore state that it is factually correct and, in most instances, you would not be able to recite this in court.

Since you attended the patient in an impartial environment, what was said at that time and recorded is part of the contemporaneous record and can be included in the statement. Although many forms of words can be used it is probably easiest to adopt a standard phrase such as 'The patient told me that' – to indicate a quote from the patient to the examining doctor.

One reason why doctors are later asked to appear in court is that there is insufficient detail in the statement so you should try to include as much detail as you feel is relevant. If the lawyers later feel that the statement contains hearsay they will remove it from the statement before presenting it to the court.

Witness Statement

(C.J. Act 1967, s9; M.C. Rules 1981, r.70)
(Magistrates Courts Act 1980 s102)

Statement of Dr John Smith *Age* over 21

This statement (consisting of ..... pages each signed by me) is true to the best of my knowledge and belief and I make it knowing that, if it is tendered in evidence, I shall be liable to prosecution if I have wilfully stated in it anything which I know to be false or do not believe to be true.

Dated .... *Signed* ....

My name is Dr Smith and I hold the Qualifications of Bachelor of Medicine and Bachelor of Surgery. On 01/04/96 during my duties as a surgical Senior House officer at Somewhere General Hospital I examined a patient Fred Jones (Date of Birth 12/03/76). He told me he had been assaulted and stabbed with a knife in the abdomen.

Examination showed that he was pale and sweaty with a pulse rate of 120 beats per minute and a blood pressure of 90/60 mmHg. His airway was clear and his heart and lungs were normal. There was an incised stab wound to his left flank below the level of his ribs (the upper part of the left hand side of his tummy) with surrounding blood. His abdomen (tummy) was tense and tender with guarding (increased muscle resistance and pain on pressing the hand into the tummy) and rebound tenderness (increasing pain when the examining hand is released from the tummy). There was an abrasion to the right side of his neck and a laceration with surrounding bruising to the back of the right hand.

Following commencement of resuscitation (giving fluids to return the pulse and blood pressure towards normal) I arranged for his transfer to theatre where I assisted Mr Singh, Consultant General Surgeon to perform an operation to explore the abdominal cavity (the inside of the tummy).

On opening the tummy there was blood within the abdomen (tummy). A probe was placed through the incised wound on the left side of the tummy from the outside and it was found that the stab wound extended through the abdominal wall and had pierced the left kidney which was the source of the bleeding within the tummy. The kidney was removed and Mr Jones' condition stabilised. The operation wound was closed and the stab wound in the side was left open on the outside although the inner layers were repaired with internal stitches. His other wounds were stitched and dressed.

He made an uneventful recovery and was discharged home well on 10/04/96. Although given an outpatient appointment on his discharge, the hospital notes record he has not returned to the outpatient department to be seen again.

Signed... *Witnessed* ....

Figure 4.2 Example of a Doctor's Statement

Present your general impression of the patient at the time (e.g.conscious/unconscious, whether the speech was slurred, if there was a smell of intoxicating liquor) and any general clinical observations performed (e.g. pulse, blood pressure, Glasgow coma score) .

If you are recording the injuries that the patient sustained, note each injury in turn using non-technical terms where possible. When this is not possible, use the correct medical term and then in parentheses add the common term which may not be absolutely accurate but will allow a lawyer to understand the injury. Record any observed negative examinations on your records (again this emphasises the importance of a full initial examination on an assault victim). Record all investigations undertaken and their results. Record any treatment given and note if any further treatment was given by other individuals who may then need to be approached for statements.

Sign at the end of the statement and then sign on each page, including the Section 9 declaration.

What should my statement *not* contain?

It is important that all words in the statement are accurate. Any impressions should be objective and not subjective. Many problems encountered with statements are due to inaccurate use of language. For example, the description given in the notes that a patient was 'drunk' is a subjective impression and can be questioned by a barrister (even the phrase 'smells of C_2H_5OH' can also be a subjective impression as pure alcohol is odour-free).

It is important to know the differences between abrasions, lacerations and incised wounds as the causation of each of these is different and can make a difference during the conduct of the case and the charges the defendant may face. Indeed, there is a specific legal definition of a wound which leads to a charge of wounding.

Do not assume any medical knowledge in those who are requesting the statement. In particular, clarify in simple English any medical terms used. Although this may not be entirely accurate in medical terms it is important for lay people to be able to understand the language. Remember that in the lay mind, there is a difference between a fracture and a broken bone.

What should a statement from another healthcare professional contain?

Most statements from other healthcare professionals are to clarify evidence or to determine an unbroken chain of evidence from a person until it is examined by a forensic scientist (e.g. a blood sample).

The introductory paragraph and Section 9 declaration (**Figure 4.1**) are the same as a Doctor's statement.

The statement then gives a record of what you did and what happened in clear, simple terms. (**Figure 4.3**).

Witness Statement

(C.J. Act 1967, s9; M.C. Rules 1981, r.70)
(Magistrates Courts Act 1980 s102)

Statement of Staff Nurse Jane Doe   *Age* over 21

This statement (consisting of ..... pages each signed by me) is true to the best of my knowledge and belief and I make it knowing that, if it is tendered in evidence, I shall be liable to prosecution if I have wilfully stated in it anything which I know to be false or do not believe to be true.

Dated ....   *Signed* ....

I am a staff nurse in the Accident & Emergency department of Somewhere General Hospital. I am a Registered General Nurse. On 01/04/96 at 22: 00 hours in the resuscitation room of the Accident & Emergency department I took a blood sample from Mr Jones and placed it in blood tubes. These were handed to the porter with instructions to take them to the on-call technician in the blood bank for urgent cross-matching.

Signed ....   *Witnessed* ....

Figure 4.3 Example of a Witness Statement

Is there anything that should *not* be in a statement made by another healthcare professional?

Do not include anything in the statment that you are not sure about. If you are unsure, say so. This is important because records of the involvement of other healthcare staff in the treatment, particularly in an emergency, are not usually formally written down in the clinical records.

As a 'witness of fact', you should not include opinion in the statement (e.g. the injuries are consistent with the history given). This is meaningless as it could also be consistent with another scenario.

What happens if the person treating the patient is not available to make the statement?

Occasionally, particularly for medical evidence, the person who treated the patient has left the hospital and cannot be traced. In these circumstances, the senior staff member on the team, while not having treated the patient, was responsible for the care they received, and may prepare the statement for the police.

In these circumstances, as well as the standard Section 9 declaration, there is another standard declaration added in the introductory part of the statement. The aim of this declaration is to show the statement was made from contemporaneous records which have not been tampered with (**Figure 4.4**).

Once again do not give an opinion as to the cause of the injuries particularly when the writer has not actually seen the patient or the injuries.

What should I do after having written a statement?

It is important that before signing any statement you read it through looking for mistakes. You need to correct simple typographical errors and ensure clarity of thought. Remember that by signing the statement you are committing yourself to the statement being true, as the declaration at the commencement of the statement indicates.

Witness Statement

(C.J. Act 1967, s9; M.C. Rules 1981, r.70)
(Magistrates Courts Act 1980 s102)

Statement of... *Age*...................

This statement (consisting of ..... pages each signed by me) is true to the best of my knowledge and belief and I make it knowing that, if it is tendered in evidence, I shall be liable to prosecution if I have wilfully stated in it anything which I know to be false or do not believe to be true.

Dated .... *Signed* ....

In connection with the making of this statement I will be referring to medical records in respect of this/these person(s).

These records are held both on a computer and on a manual record system held by the Hospital. The records held on both the computer and manual system were created by persons/employees in the course of the business of the Hospital, and the information contained and the information obtained in these records was supplied by employees who had, or may reasonably be supposed to have had, personal knowledge of the matters dealt with.

To the best of my knowledge and belief there are no reasonable grounds for believing that the information in the records is inaccurate, because of improper use: At all material times the computer was operating properly, or if not, any respect in which it was not operating properly, or was out of operation was not such as to affect the production of the information or the accuracy of its contents.

Figure 4.4 Example of Declaration regarding notes.

If you are happy that the contents of the statement are correct, sign and submit the statement to the requesting police officer.

Can I charge for the time taken to prepare a statement?

Doctors providing statements are acting as professional witnesses and as such can claim a standard fee for the provision of the medical statement. Most police forces have a standard form which has multiple copies to be sent both to the officer requesting the statement and the finance department of the police force for processing.

What happens if the statement is not clear or the police have other specific questions?

Sometimes, after a statement has been prepared, the police return to the writer asking for clarification of a medical term. In these circumstances, a simple addendum to the statement clarifying the point may be all that is necessary (and a mental note to make the original statement clearer if asked for another statement).

Sometimes, however, the police may ask specific questions. This is probably due to the defence having served evidence that disputes the medical evidence and the police may be asking for an explanation as to the cause of the wounds. If you feel confident that you can give an explanation or there is evidence that an explanation does not fit with the recorded medical facts, you can give a further statement answering the specific questions asked by the police.

It is best to return both the questions you have been asked and your answers in the statement so that the police can see clearly exactly what you have answered.

Do the police have any rights to interview patients in hospital?

The police sometimes wish to interview patients who are in hospital undergoing treatment. They may also wish the patient to provide specimens, particularly after road traffic accidents. This is done, not by the treating doctor but, by a police surgeon (also called a forensic medical examiner).

Before the patient is approached to provide a sample, the police must gain consent from the doctor treating the patient. When consent has been given, the police may interview the patient and subsequently ask him or her to provide a sample.

What happens if the patient is clinically unwell ?

If the treating doctor feels that an interview or the provision of a sample would worsen the clinical condition of the patient (e.g. providing a breath sample in a patient with a chest injury) they may refuse the police the right to obtain such a specimen.

Can the police obtain a specimen without the consent of the patient ?

As well as deciding that the clinical condition of the patient will not worsen because of an approach by the police, the doctor must also be convinced that the patient can understand the request to provide a sample and can give informed consent to such a request.

Occasionally, the defence in such cases looks for inappropriate use of this consent. Therefore, it is vital to remember that all notes made prior to the request and the subsequent treatment of the patient may be important in determining the validity of the police involvement. This means that in addition to not making the patient worse by the request, the doctor must be convinced that there is no reason for the patient not to understand the request. Failure to provide a specimen in such circumstances is in itself an offence and the penalty can be as severe as that given for driving with alcohol in the blood.

Are there any circumstances where the rights of a patient can be overruled?

In the case of a serious offence, particularly terrorism, there may be a duty, although not an obligation, to allow police access without consent. In these particular narrow circumstances, the healthcare professional should seek advice both from within their place of employment and from their defence organisation before taking this step.

Can the patient challenge the consent process?

Patients can obtain access, under the Access to Health records Act 1990, to their clinical records. This may lead to the clinical condition of the patient as recorded in the notes being reviewed by an independent doctor advising the patient in subsequent proceedings and the records will have critical importance to that assessment.

It is therefore important to document the clinical state of the patient as this may again be relevant in subsequent treatment.

Expert witness in criminal cases

What happens if the defendant disputes the medical evidence?

In many cases, there is dispute as to the cause of specific injuries. This may be due to the differences between the accounts given by the complainant (the injured party) and the assailant to their respective legal teams.

In these cases, an independent professional may be asked to give expert advice as to the cause of injuries.

How can the expert evidence be provided?

If the defence legal team feel that there is sufficient doubt as to the cause of injuries, and differing explanations of the force involved in those injuries, they may approach an independent medical practitioner to review the medical evidence in the case.

How does a solicitor find such an individual?

Most solicitors find their expert witnesses through a variety of sources. Some are recommended by other practising solicitors and barristers who have seen the healthcare professional provide evidence before (this may not necessarily be as a criminal expert witness). A number of organisations produce registers of healthcare professionals willing to give expert advice on such matters. Individuals may also advertise their services in legal publications. Finally, there are organisations for expert witnesses who can provide a search facility to a solicitor with a individual problem (see **Appendix D**).

What happens when a solicitor identifies a possible expert?

Having found the name of a possible expert, the solicitor will approach that individual either by letter (Figure 4.5) or telephone. These letters are often sent without a preceding telephone call.

Jones & Sons
Solicitors
1 High Street
Anytown

Mr G Smythe
Consultant Surgeon
Nowhere City Hospital

Dear Sirs

re Regina vs. John Smith

We represent the defendant in the above case who is charged with malicious wounding of another person.

Our client maintains that during an argument the complainant fell against a knife protruding from the edge of a kitchen unit and thus sustained the injury to his abdomen.

We write to ask if you would be prepared to review the medical evidence in this case and provide us with a report regarding your view as to the cause of the injuries sustained.

We have in our possession statements from the doctors who treated the patient together with the statements of our client and the complainant and photographs of the crime scene. The knife is in the possession of the CPS and would be available for inspection by arrangement.

Our case is liable to be listed for hearing at Crown Court within the next 3 months and your report would be needed within the next 6 weeks.

We have to obtain prior authority from the Legal Aid board to incur this expense and would be grateful if you could submit an estimate of the likely cost (both the total cost and your hourly rate) for the preparation of such a report

If you are willing to assist us in this matter we would appreciate a speedy response when we will send a fuller letter of instruction together with the documents we have available

Yours faithfully

Figure 4.5 Example of a letter of instruction

What do I do if I receive such a letter?

If you are approached as an expert witness in criminal cases it is important, as in all expert appointments, to consider whether you are the most appropriate person to prepare the report. Many lawyers do not have an intimate knowledge of the specialisms within medicine or the qualifications of other healthcare professionals with regard to such matters.

It is also wise to consider, particularly in criminal cases, whether there is any conflict of interest (i.e. if the patient has been treated by a close colleague or within your hospital).

Most requests will be specific about the questions the solicitor wishes you to answer, but as with all independent expert advice your duty is to examine all of the relevant evidence before giving an opinion.

What do I do if I wish to prepare the report?

If you feel you are able and willing to prepare the report, you should send the solicitor a letter confirming your willingness and setting out your terms and conditions for preparing the report (**Figure 4.6**). If they agree to these terms they will acknowledge your letter and send you what they feel to be all relevant documentation.

Dear Sirs

re Regina vs. **Smith**

Thank you for your letter. Based on the information in your initial letter I feel able to assist you in providing a report on the medical evidence in this case.

My fees based on the information given would be around £400 based on an hourly rate of £100. At present this is an estimate without seeing the documents and if the work on inspection of these documents is likely to exceed this figure I will inform you prior to commencing the preparation of the report. I will also invoice you for any expenses and provide receipts for such expenses

On receipt of your full instructions and the relevant documents I will be able to prepare a report within 4 weeks and will deliver it with my invoice at that time.

My standard terms are 60 days for payment of the invoice from presentation.

I will use my experience, care and skill in fulfilling your instructions to the best of my ability.

Yours faithfully

Figure 4.6 Reply to solicitors letter

What happens next?

On receipt of the letter, the solicitor will normally issue fuller instructions and enclose the material they have available.

Dear Sir

Thank you for your letter. We have obtained authority from the Legal Aid Board to obtain a report at a cost not exceeding £400.

Our client was the previous boyfriend of Miss James who now resides with the complainant, Mr Jones. Our client and this young woman have a son and recently he has been pursued for the support of that child.

He went to her flat on the night of the incident to discuss both access to their son and payment of support and he alleges he was confronted by Mr Jones (who now lives in the flat) who told him that Miss James did not wish him to see the boy.

Our client alleges that a heated argument took place and that Mr Jones attacked him. While trying to get out of the flat he admits punching Mr Jones causing him to fall against a protruding knife. Mr Jones alleges that our client deliberately found the knife and stabbed him.

Our purpose in commissioning a report is to ask you to examine the evidence and give an opinion as to whether either or both of the accounts given of the incident can account for the injuries that Mr Jones sustained.

We enclose the following documents

Statement from Dr Smith, Senior House Officer in Surgery

Statement from Mr Singh, Consultant General Surgeon.

Statement of Dr Gray, Police Surgeon who examined our client while in custody.

Statement of PC White regarding the premises and photographs of the house.

Statement of Mr Jones.

Transcript of recorded interviews with our client.

Our client's proof of evidence.

Please do not consider this list exhaustive and if you feel that there is any other information that may help in formulating the report, please do not hesitate to contact the writer of this letter.

In criminal cases the burden of proof is beyond reasonable doubt and I must ask you to remember this when preparing your report.

We will need to serve your report on the prosecution in statement form and we should be grateful if you could type at the start as follows

Statement of.. *Age*................

This statement (consisting of ..... pages each signed by me) is true to the best of my knowledge and belief and I make it knowing that, if it is tendered in evidence, I shall be liable to prosecution if I have wilfully stated in it anything which I know to be false or do not believe to be true.

Dated .... *Signed* ....

Please also sign each page of your statement.

Yours faithfully

Figure 4.7 Sample letter

What documents should I examine?

As an expert witness, the report should be based on *all* relevant evidence. With luck, the instructing solicitor will have given you all the papers they have, including witness statements.

This includes any evidence to be used in court and, if possible, original material such as hospital records and X-rays which may be relevant. However, disclosure of the medical records of a third party may not be given as that patient has a right to withhold consent to release these records.

In many cases therefore, not all the records are obtained and, if the healthcare professional preparing the report feels that there is missing evidence which may influence their opinion they should discuss this matter with their instructing solicitor at the earliest opportunity.

If, despite this, these documents are still not available for the preparation of the report, this should be made clear in the introduction to the report.

It is clear that not only should clinical records be available, but also witness statements and, quite possibly, a statement from the client concerned.

What format should the report take?

As this report is being prepared for criminal proceedings it is easier if a similar format to a witness statement is used. The 'Section 9 declaration' (**Figure 4.1**) should appear on the front page and each subsequent page should be signed.

All documents studied should be listed, as should any documents known to exist, but which have not been made available for inspection.

The clinical evidence should be set out with particular reference to any photographic or other evidence available.

A summary of the accounts contained in the witness statements, where relevant to the questions you have been asked to give an opinion on, should be set out.

How should I present my opinion?

The burden of proof in a criminal case is that of 'beyond reasonable doubt'. This must be remembered when preparing your opinion.

The best starting point is the clinical evidence. Using your experience, how could those injuries have been caused?

Having decided this in isolation, consider then the varying accounts of how the injuries are alleged to have been caused. If one explanation is completely inconsistent with the medical evidence then state this.

Is more than one explanation possible? Indicate any alternative explanations for the injuries. If one explanation is more likely to have caused the injuries than another, then explain this, giving your clinical reasons for preferring the explanation given in *your* report.

Remember that this report is prepared for the court. Your opinion on the evidence is based solely on the evidence present, not on the 'side' which has given you instructions.

You may consider that both accounts given of the cause of the injuries are consistent with the injuries themselves. It is not your job to decide which account is to be believed. This will be a matter for the jury at the trial.

What should I do having prepared the report?

Having prepared the report, read it through and confirm that each part of your opinion can be justified by the factual evidence you have been given. Then, sign every page of the report and the Section 9 declaration and send it to the solicitor with a separate fee note.

What happens if further evidence is produced?

If, after the report is prepared, further statements or medical evidence are forthcoming read these critically. If these make you alter your opinion then do so, as these are facts which you will be shown in court. If, however, they only add a further alternative explanation to the cause of the injuries and do not change the opinions on the facts you had previously studied, then it is proper to make this known to your instructing solicitor. Only when the facts are decided can your opinion be valid.

Check list for police statement

Before starting

- Did I have contact with the patient?
- Am I disclosing clinical details?
- Is there consent for disclosure?
- Do I have the original notes and X-rays?

Making the statement

- Have I given my name and qualifications?
- Have I identified the patient using their name and date of birth?
- Have I described the history they gave?
- Have I explained each injury in non-technical terms?
- Have I described my involvement and the limits of my knowledge?

After making the statement

- Have I read the statement for errors and corrected them?
- Have I read and signed the 'Section 9 Declaration' on the front page?
- Have I signed each page of the statement?
- Have I kept my own copy of the statement and copies of the relevant notes ?
- Have I completed any claim form for payment?
- Has the statement been sent to the appropriate authorities?

Check list for expert report in criminal cases

On receiving initial approach

- Does the letter indicate that the questions being asked are appropriate to my expertise?
- Have I treated the patient/know the treating doctor well?
- Can I complete the investigation and report in the time allowed?
- Am I prepared to act?

Terms and conditions

- Are my terms clear and the cost both in time and money detailed?
- Are my terms accepted in full?

Before preparing report

- Having seen the full instructions, is my fee still reasonable?
- Am I the right person to prepare this report?
- Are the original notes/X-rays available or are there only statements/copies?
- Are witness statements enclosed?
- Are crime scene photographs enclosed?
- Are transcripts enclosed?

The report

- Have I summarised the medical evidence clearly in simple language?
- Have I taken each of the explanations and given an opinion of them related to the medical evidence?
- Are my conclusions clear?

After preparing the report

- Have I checked the report for clarity and errors?
- Have I signed the 'Section 9 declaration' on the front page?
- Have I signed each page of the report?
- Have I kept a copy of the report?
- Have I enclosed my fee note with the report?

5

Criminal court oral evidence

Aims

This chapter will help you

- To understand the structure of criminal courts in England & Wales

- To prepare to give evidence in the Criminal Courts

- To understand the differences between a professional and expert witness in the criminal court

Criminal cases in England are decided in the Criminal courts. There are two layers of this system for the trial; the Magistrates Court and the Crown Court.

What is a Magistrates court?

A Magistrates Court is the court where all criminal offences are initially heard. Some offences are dealt with here and sentence is passed. Other offences may need to be decided in Crown Court. The evidence gathered is initially presented in a Magistrates Court and, if there is a substantial case made on the evidence, the case will be sent ('committed') for a full trial at Crown Court.

Who arranges for witnesses to appear in Magistrates Court?

If you are required to appear in the Magistrates Court you are likely to be contacted by the administrative support unit of the local police force who will inform you of the date, time and place of the court hearing. In some instances, this may be the day prior to the hearing and often you are only given the name of the defendant in the case.

This may be of little help if you did not examine the defendant but the injured party. Unless you specifically request the name of the patient on whom you prepared a statement, you will spend many fruitless hours looking for your statement.

Having found out the name of the patient you examined, search for all the medical records on that patient. Do not leave this until the day before the hearing or you may discover that records are not in file and this is guaranteed to increase your stress level. Collect all the notes and any X-rays along with your copy of the statement.

What to do when you arrive at court?

Always anticipate that the journey to court will take double the time it would normally. It is always better to arrive early and be able to sit quietly rather than to be rushing in just on time, and having to appear in the witness box while still recovering from your journey. Such a state of mind is not conducive to clear thought.

On arrival at the court building, find out which court you are attending and where it is located. Introduce yourself to the list calling officer or the usher of the court who will hold the list of witnesses for each individual case.

If you are not asked directly about taking the oath, inform the usher or list calling officer which holy book you wish to use to take the oath or whether you wish to affirm. Most courts now have the holy books available for the majority of religions.

Ask for the legal representative for the CPS who is likely to have requested your presence because you initially made the statement for the police. In the Magistrates Court this is more likely to be a solicitor than a barrister.

You may have time to sit down quietly and review both the medical records and the statement you have prepared. While you may refer to the medical records in the witness box you will not normally be allowed access to your statement. If you have not been to a court before, ask to look into the court before the case starts, to familarise yourself with the layout of the court.

Once the case has started, 'witnesses of fact', including professional witnesses, are not allowed to be present in the court.

Having reviewed these records you will probably have some time to wait. Do not allow yourself to get frustrated during this time as this will only impede your performance in the witness box. Make sure you take something to read or work on while you are waiting.

Who decides cases in the Magistrates Court?

Cases are heard by magistrates who may either be qualified and paid (stipendiary magistrates) or voluntary lay magistrates appointed by the Lord Chancellor. A stipendiary magistrate can sit alone but lay magistrates normally number three in a court. In addition, the magistrates are advised on the law by a Clerk to the Justices.

What happens when I am called to give evidence?

When you are required in court, the clerk will call your name and direct you into court and to the witness box. Remember to take all original notes with you and ensure that any other possessions are safe.

What happens on entering the witness box?

When you first enter the witness box you will take the oath. This will normally be printed on a card and you will be asked to hold the Bible, or other holy book, in your right hand. If you have no religious belief you can elect to affirm.

In both cases, the evidence presented after having made either an oath or affirmation is the same and carries the same weight and responsibilities.

Evidence in Chief

After taking the oath, you will initially be questioned by the party who requested your attendance at court.

You will first be asked your name and professional address (it is probably wise not to give your home address when called as a professional witness to court). You may be asked to give your qualifications and your appointment (both the one you now hold and the one you held at the time of the relevant incident).

You may be asked to relate your involvement with the patient and, in most cases, will be allowed to refer to notes made at the time of the incident.

During this time, answer only the question that is asked and do not try to guess what the next question will be. Explain any technical terms either with a verbal description or by pointing to the appropriate part of your own body. If you do not understand a question, ask for it to be repeated.

The questions during examination in chief cannot be leading questions (i.e. questions that suggest an answer by the witness). If the opposing lawyer feels that the question is a leading question he will ask for the question to be rephrased.

For example the lawyer cannot ask you on examination in chief 'the patient was unsteady was he?' but he can ask 'what did you observe on initially seeing the patient'?

What is cross-examination?

The purpose of cross-examination is for the opposing lawyer to test the evidence you have given to the court.

After giving your evidence to the lawyer for the party who called you, the lawyer for the other party will ask you questions. If you have given your statement as a professional witness you are appearing in court as a 'witness of fact' and, as such, should not be drawn into giving opinions. If the lawyer continues to try and make you give an opinion, decide whether you are qualified to give one or not, answer truthfully if you do not have the experience to give an opinion and, in most cases, the magistrates will accept this and stop the questioning. If you do wish to give an opinion and are qualified to do so, you may ask the Magistrates if they wish to treat you as an expert witness.

During cross-examination, leading questions can be asked and should be answered truthfully but if more than a simple yes/no answer is needed, do not be afraid to expand, even if the lawyer who asked the question attempts to stop anything other than a single word answer.

What is re-examination?

After you have been cross-examined, the lawyer who initially called you may ask further questions to clarify points raised by his opponent in the cross-examination. If you have been asked to consider one scenario by the cross-examiner which would fit with his case, the other lawyer may offer an alternative for you to consider.

Can anyone else ask me questions apart from the lawyers?

The magistrates may ask questions to clarify points they do not understand. This may occur during your answers to the lawyers or after the lawyers have completed their questions.

Where should my answers be directed?

Remember that the decision on the case is being made by the magistrates, not the lawyer who is questioning you. Your answers should therefore be addressed to the bench (the place where the magistrates are sitting).

How fast should I speak?

As the evidence is presented in court, it is written down (often still in long hand) by a clerk and/or by the magistrates themselves. You should therefore watch and pause during your answers to allow those writing your replies to keep up.

Remember that lawyers who are more used to the environment will be watching the transcription and may pause after you have completed your answer before asking a further question.

The flow of the questions and answers may appear stilted at times but it is crucial for the evidence to be correctly transcribed during these proceedings.

What happens after I have completed my evidence?

If the case is being tried in the Magistrates Court and the decision will be made in there, the court, mindful of the pressures on healthcare professionals, will normally release them quickly. The magistrates will also warn the healthcare professional that as a condition of release, they must not speak to anyone yet to give evidence about the trial or about their own evidence.

If the case is being heard at the Magistrates court before being sent for trial at the Crown Court and the healthcare professional has given evidence, the court may wish to avoid this evidence being presented in oral form again at Crown Court and may have the evidence presented as a written statement to the higher court.

In such cases, the evidence presented will be transcribed into a written format which can be presented in the Crown Court. This must be checked and signed by the witness as a true record both of the questions asked and the answers given before the witness is released from the court.

Can I claim a fee for attending court?

If you appear as a witness in court you are entitled to your expenses, including loss of earnings. In addition, professional witnesses can claim a fee for the time they were absent from work to be in court. These fees are paid by the court and a claim form should be completed before leaving the court.

Can I use the courtroom experience as a learning tool?

It may well be a valuable exercise to review your performance in court and use it as a learning tool.

It may also be that the learning point is not your performance in the witness box, but the contents of the statement you prepared which has led to your appearance in court. A suggested debriefing checklist appears at the end of this chapter.

What is a witness order?

If you have given a statement, it is likely to be presented as evidence in committal proceedings without requiring your presence. During the committal proceedings the evidence to be used in Crown Court is disclosed and the persons making those statements are normally given witness orders. (**Figure 5.1**)

If the evidence is likely to be accepted by both sides (and in most cases the details of the injuries are likely to be) the healthcare professional will be given a conditional witness order. If questions are likely to be asked about the evidence then an unconditional order will be made.

What should I do if I receive a witness order ?

Having received a witness order, it is important to note that there are penalties attached to the order if you fail to attend the court if called to give evidence.

It is also likely that there will be some time between the committal proceedings, at which the witness order has been made, and the trial. During that time, many healthcare professionals may change jobs and even move away from the hospital where they were working when they prepared the initial statement.

It is, therefore, good practice to inform the listing officer for the court of any future plans to move away from your current address held on file and also to give the listing officer some indication of any prior commitments that you may have in the 6 months following the witness order. It is important to always quote the court reference number when sending any communication to the court regarding your witness order. If the witness order does not give the name of the patient for whom you prepared the statement, it is also important to obtain this information from the court office when confirming your availability.

St. Elsewhere Police

Criminal Justice Unit
St. Elsewhere Police Station
St. Elsewhere
XX22 DD33

Dr W. Blogg
C/O Healthcare NHS Trust
Accident & Emergency Dept
St. Elsewhere

Direct Line:
Tel:
Fax:

Date:
Please ask for: Witness Liaison Officer

Please quote this reference number:

WITNESS WARNING NOTICE

Dear ....
Ref: R v ....
You should have received from us information explaining that court proceedings have started in the above case and you may be required to give evidence as a witness.

The Crown Prosecution Service have told us that you are required and the hearing is scheduled to take place as indicated below.

Time	TWO pm
Date	Monday 01/01/98
Court	St. Elsewhere Crown Court, Law Courts, St. Elsewhere

Please complete and return the reply slip below <u>as soon as possible</u>, in the envelope provided (Freepost: no stamp required).

Please note that if you do not attend, without good reason, the court may issue a summons or warrant compelling your attendance. Therefore, if you experience any difficulties or find yourself unable to attend you must contact the Witness Liaison Officer on the above number without delay. To help us process your enquiry promptly please quote the reference number.

We enclose a Witness in Court Booklet and information to assist your attendance. **Please bring this letter with you to court as it will assist the court usher to help with your visit.** Should you require further help please do not hesitate to contact us.

Yours sincerely

Chief Inspector, Criminal Justice Unit
DETACH HERE AND RETAIN ABOVE FOR YOUR INFORMATION
....

Please sign and return this slip
Reference number:

Time	Two pm	
Date	Monday 01/01/98	
Court	St. Elsewhere Magistrates Court	

Ms. M Private
Criminal Justice Unit
St Elsewhere Police Station

From: Dr W Blogg
C/O Healthcare NHS Trust
Accident & Emergency Dept
St Elsewhere

Telephone Home:
Telephone Works:

Figure 5.1 Example witness order

When will the trial date be arranged?

Initially, the court will arrange a trial date. At this time, the administrative support unit of the police may call you asking for specific commitments not already notified to them over a shorter period of time.

The court will then arrange a trial date for the Crown court and will notify you of the date for the hearing.

This may either be a definite date for the commencement of the trial or the trial could be placed on a list of trials arranged to occur at some time during a particular week depending on time in the courts. This is called the 'warned list'. Sometimes these dates are changed or moved to another 'warned list' depending on changes in court circumstances or changes in the case itself.

If the latter occurs, the exact day of the trial may only be known the day before it is due to commence and may not even be known until the evening of the previous day. It is therefore important if the exact date of a trial is not known but you have been called as a witness to begin your preparations early.

What happens if I have commitments on the day or week of the hearing?

In most cases, the court will take note of the professionals' commitments but may ask how fixed these commitments are.

If the court decides that the case will go ahead they will subpoena the healthcare professional and there are severe penalties if he/she does not attend the court.

What do I do when the date of the court is fixed and I am aware of the day?

The main priority when the date is fixed is to prepare all the clinical records available on the patient and ensure they are in a safe place before the day of the case. This is especially important if you have left the institution where you prepared the report as you will have to rely on someone from the medical records department to prepare the records for you to collect prior to attending the court.

You should also find and review the contents of the statement you prepared. It is also important that you find out from the solicitor who has called you if they wish you to arrive at a particular time before proceedings begin in order to have a conference with the barrister.

What to do on the day of the hearing

On the day of the hearing, arrive at the court in plenty of time. Expect that the journey will take double the time that it would normally take and expect that there will be no parking places.

It is better to spend some time sitting in the court than to arrive after the court proceedings have commenced as you may be faced with entering the witness box immediately.

Who to see when you arrive

When you arrive in court you should look on the court listing indicating which court the case is being held in and then approach the usher supervising that court and confirm your presence. In addition, ask that the solicitor who has asked for your appearance be informed of your arrival.

Who will be in charge of the conduct of the case in court?

In the Crown Court, the case is normally conducted by a barrister although some solicitors now have rights of audience in Crown Court. Before the case commences, it is worthwhile asking the solicitor for a conference with the advocate, and indeed most advocates will want to discuss the case with the healthcare professional and may also be able to give you some idea why the clinical evidence contained in your statement has not been accepted without your appearance in court.

What happens when the case starts?

Although the courts are mindful of the commitments of healthcare professionals outside court, and try to inconvenience them as little as possible, there is no point in presenting the clinical evidence in court without having established the factual background of the case. This means that other 'witnesses of fact' are likely to be called before the healthcare professional and there may be some time to wait.

During this wait, which may appear much longer than it is in reality, do not become frustrated as it may then be apparent when you enter the witness box. The impression you would then give is not what you would prefer and may give the jury a false impression of the evidence you present.

Once again, remember to take something to work on or read.

Is there anything else that I need to do before being called to give evidence?

As the first thing you will be asked to do on entering the witness box is to take the oath, it is important that the clerk of the court is aware of the holy book you wish to use to take the oath. If that holy book is not available you may have to affirm.

What happens when I am called to give evidence?

When your name is called you will be ushered into the witness box by a court official. You will then be asked to take the oath and should recite this in an ordinary voice neither being over-confident nor flippant. Use this time to familiarise yourself with the layout of the court. (**Figure 5.2**)

Whom am I addressing?

You should address the jury and the judge. They are often at a different angle to the barristers asking the questions.

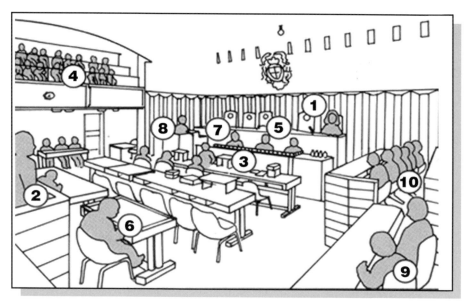

Figure 5.2 Diagram of a typical courtroom at the Central Criminal Court, the Old Bailey.
1 Judge.   2 Accused.   3 Counsel.   4 Public gallery.   5 Court clerk.   6 Solicitors.
7 Shorthand writer.   8 Witness box.   9 Press.   10 Jury.

You should stand facing the jury, then turn your body towards the barrister to allow him to ask a question. When answering the question, you should turn back to face the jury. Then turn back to the barrister when you have finished answering the question. This will allow you to avoid the barrister's techniques, such as rustling papers or appearing disinterested while you are answering.

What details about myself should I give as a professional witness?

As a professional witness, your qualifications and experience will normally be requested by the barrister, as will your current employment and the job you were in when the statement was prepared (should this be different). If requested, give the hospital address. Do not use your home address.

The barrister will take you through your evidence as given on your statement. You will not have this statement in the witness box but should have the original medical records to which you can refer if you ask the judge.

When answering the questions, do not use technical terms. Use simple English and remember to use your own body to point out the location of injuries to help the jury understand the position of anatomical locations used in the notes.

Having taken you through the evidence in the statement, you may find that the barrister asks you for an opinion as to the cause of the injuries. While you may give an opinion by way of an explanation, remember not to overstep the mark that your experience dictates and if you cannot give an opinion tell the barrister that it is outside your area of expertise.

In cross-examination by the opposing barrister, you are likely to find not only the injuries that have been recorded in your statement questioned but possibly other negative findings. Remember when writing clinical notes therefore to look for, and record, all important negative findings.

If the clinical records do not show anything, say so and if you cannot remember, be truthful. Sometimes it may feel like you are the one on trial but remember you are only a witness.

Who else can ask questions?

The judge may ask for clarification during the questioning. One or other of the barristers can ask supplementary questions at the end of the evidence heard from both barristers. The jury may also send notes to the judge asking for clarification if they feel that an answer is unclear and the judge may ask the witness about these concerns on behalf of the jury.

At what speed should I answer questions?

The judge is taking notes of your answers to the questions in longhand (although some courts have now invested in new technology). Watch the judge and do not rush through your answers. In most cases, the barrister will wait for the judge before asking the next question. If you rush ahead the judge may ask you to slow down. In addition, the evidence may be taped and transcribed contemporaneously by a stenographer.

What happens after the questions have been asked?

Having given your evidence, the court normally allows you to be released to return to your normal duties. If the court extends this privilege to you then it is important that you do not discuss the evidence you have given with anyone else who is yet to give evidence.

Can I claim for attending court?

Witnesses can claim their expenses and healthcare professionals called as professional witnesses can elect to have a witness fee paid instead of loss of earnings. It is important to obtain this form and submit it to the court as quickly as possible following attendance at court.

Should I formally appraise my performance after the court appearance?

Every experience, both good and bad, can be used to influence future behaviour. Although your instinct may be to get away from court and forget about the experience, quiet reflection both on the questions asked in court and the reason for your appearance can help you to understand the reason why your statement was not accepted as evidence without your attendance.

You may learn the importance of noting negative findings or looking for other types of injuries. You may also learn that while the length of a wound may be irrelevant in clinical practice, it may be important to the legal process as is the number of stitches inserted in a wound.

You may find that you enjoy the forensic aspects of the healthcare professional's life and this could influence your future career or interests.

A checklist to help with this is provided as a guide at the end of this chapter.

The expert witness in Crown Court

If a healthcare professional has been asked to give an expert opinion in a criminal case and has prepared a report, it is likely that he or she will be called to court if this opinion offers an alternative explanation for the injuries, casting reasonable doubt on the charges which someone faces.

It is often the case that the clinical evidence has been prepared from medical records and that an opinion has not been sought from the professional witness who prepared that statement. Indeed the statement may have been made by a relatively junior clinician who does not have the necessary experience to make such a judgment.

Having prepared a statement, the healthcare professional acting in an expert capacity may be asked for their time commitments to prepare for a trial in the court.

While 'witnesses of fact' cannot avoid attending court, even if it is inconvenient, an expert witness can only be compelled to attend on a specific day if a subpoena has been granted. Most solicitors are unwilling to do this as an expert witness who is forced to attend court may be unwilling to give an opinion in a future case for these solicitors. It is unfortunate that many experts react very strongly to a subpoena because the solicitors are simply trying to do their job – to ensure a smooth trial. In addition, if an expert is very busy, it is important for the firm who subpeona'd him that the expert will appear. This may be to the detriment of the future clients of the solicitor.

It is therefore important to keep in touch with the solicitor and to reply promptly to any letter asking for the suitability of a court date (**Figure 5.3**).

Dear Sirs

re Regina vs Minot

We write further to your report on the medical evidence in the above case. We have served your report as a statement but as yet the Crown Prosecution Service has not indicated that it is willing to accept your evidence and at present we require you to give evidence on our client's behalf.

The trial is at present in the warned list for the week beginning 2/9/98 and has been listed for 2 days. We cannot at present determine which days you will be required as this may not be fixed until the day before the trial commences due to other trials occurring.

We therefore ask you to write confirming that you are available throughout that week or informing us of any time during that week when you could not attend court. If there is no suitable time that you could attend that week we will apply for an adjournment but would require dates during the next 3 months when you would be available so as to gain a fixture in the court listing for this matter.

We would be grateful for an indication of the fee you would charge for attendance at court being mindful that the Criminal Legal Aid fund imposes maximum fees for expert witnesses which are only rarely exceeded.

Yours faithfully

Solicitors

Figure 5.3 Example letter

How should the expert prepare for court?

Just as the professional witness to the court prepares for court, the expert witness should do the same. In serious cases, this may include a conference with the barrister conducting the case prior to the court date.

It is important, however, even if the conference is not arranged, that all the evidence the expert has used in the preparation of the report, and the report itself, should be re-examined prior to attendance at court.

It is also proper that the expert should make the solicitor aware both of his availability and of the fees he intends to charge. These should be agreed by the solicitor (if not done already). This may require prior approval by the legal aid board.

If the expert feels that clinical evidence which he has not seen may be important to the opinion he has given (and has stated that in his report) he should make the solicitor aware of any primary clinical records he wishes to have in court if he does not have copies of them to hand. If you are acting on behalf of the Defendant, clinical records for the victim will only be released through the Crown Prosecution Service with the victim's consent. If this consent is not given, the only way these will be released is by order of the judge. They will then be available at court.

It is also vital if the court is unknown to the expert that he or she asks for details regarding location, appropriate parking or accommodation if required (**Figure 5.4**).

If you have never given evidence before or feel you could learn more with some practise, consider attending courtroom skills training (See Appendix D).

What to do on the day of the trial?

On the day of the trial, the expert witness may meet the barrister conducting the case in conference at court

---

Dear Sirs

re Regina vs Minot

Thank you for your letter regarding the trial dates for the above case. I am available throughout that week apart from the Wednesday when I have clinical commitments which cannot be altered.

I have as yet not seen the CT scan of Mr Singh which was performed in St Otherwise Infirmary and I feel that it is vital to my opinion that this is available in court on the day of the hearing.

My fees for attendance are £250 for preparation for trial and £450 per day or part thereof spent in court. In addition, expenses incurred will be charged.

I would be grateful for directions by train to the court and the time you wish me to arrive on the day of the hearing. While I accept the unpredictable nature of such hearings I would appreciate as much notice as possible.

Yours faithfully

Mr A Cannon
Consultant Surgeon

Figure 5.4 Example letter

prior to the commencement of proceedings. At this conference, the barrister and the expert should discuss the strengths and weaknesses of the clinical evidence and the opinion the expert has given.

If further evidence has been made available since the expert made their initial report, this should also be examined.

What differences are there between an expert and professional witness?

Because an expert witness is giving an opinion on the facts she is entitled to hear the facts of the case. Therefore, unlike other witnesses who cannot sit in the court until after they have given evidence, the expert witness can sit in the court chamber and listen to the evidence being presented during the trial.

The expert is independent of the case and primarily there to help the court understand technical issues.

Expert witnesses normally sit behind the barrister with the solicitor for whom they prepared the report.

During the conference and whilst the evidence is being presented and tested by examination and cross-examination, the expert must keep an open mind on the opinion she has given. If the factual evidence changes during the trial resulting in the expert changing the opinion given in her report she should inform the barrister immediately both of the nature and the reasons for this change.

Should the expert provide advice to the barrister during the trial?

Often during the trial, clinical evidence will be presented either in written or oral form. If the expert has prepared a report questioning the cause of specific injuries, the doctor who examined the victim and who prepared a statement, may appear as a witness in the court.

The expert should listen attentively, looking for evidence not present in the clinical notes or other clinical material not previously disclosed. If such material is presented, it is important that the barrister asks if his expert could examine this evidence. The trial may be adjourned to allow this to take place.

If the defence has an alternative explanation for the cause of specific injuries which has been confirmed in the expert report, the barrister may ask the professional witness if that could indeed be a cause of the injuries the expert has observed.

If you wish to pass a note to the barrister during the proceedings, write it down on a pad of paper and pass it forward while the witness is still in the witness box. Make sure the barrister can clearly read the note and put the time the note was made on the piece of paper. If it is of vital importance, he may turn to the expert witness and ask a further question in light of the note. Before the case, confirm with the barrister the form he wishes notes to take.

If the professional witness answers unexpectedly, the barrister may turn to you and ask if the statement the witness has made is correct.

What does an expert witness have to establish in the witness box?

To present expert evidence, the healthcare professional must establish themselves as an expert in the eyes of the court before they can give opinion evidence.

This normally means that, in addition to their professional qualifications, their experience must be established to the satisfaction of the court.

Experience is normally established by the barrister after the expert witness has taken the oath or affirmed.

Although called by one party to the proceedings the expert witness has a duty solely to the court.

Remember that as an expert you are not there to determine the facts of the case. That is the role of the jury.

If two accounts of the same incident are equally plausible as explanations for a group of injuries, it is not for the expert to say which account is correct. He or she can only say that the injuries could have been caused by either method, that one explanation is more likely than the other and can give his/her reasons for that opinion.

As the report is evidence the expert has prepared prior to the court appearance, the report is normally brought out during examination in chief, by the barrister acting for the party that has called the expert.

Remember that when the evidence was given to you, it was in the form of statements and not all the witness statements provided may have been available to the expert at the time of preparing the report. This will be evident because the expert will be present in court as the 'witnesses of fact' give their evidence.

If the facts change and you are asked in the witness box about a set of facts you had not previously considered, it is important to ask for time to consider these so that you can give an accurate answer.

While you may have access to any relevant papers you had in your possession after having entered the witness box, you may have no communication with the barrister or solicitor who called you but must rely on your own sources of information.

Cross-examination of an expert witness

As an expert witness, the cross-examination is likely not only to question your evidence but also you and your qualifications to give that evidence. This is done to undermine the credibility of the witness and therefore the evidence they have given.

This may include asking questions outside the field of your expertise or asking a series of simple questions in sequence: each in themselves are simple to answer but the end result may be that a position established at the beginning is completely reversed by the end.

If the prosecution gives many different scenarios to you asking for opinions, give each careful thought before confirming or denying the possible truth of the scenarios.

What to do after giving evidence

Expert evidence is normally given near the conclusion of a trial after all factual evidence has been presented.

Normally, therefore, the court will release the expert after they have given evidence.

As an expert witness you can claim a fee for attending court and for the preparation time taken for the case. This is paid out of criminal court funds and the solicitor will normally have the form available. If you have given notice of fees prior to attendance and these have been agreed, it is important to note this on the claim form.

Checklists for professional witnesses

Magistrates Court

Name of patient

Trial name

Court ref

Date of trial

Place of trial

Medical records obtained

Copy statement

Witness order

Court ref

Patient name

Availability confirmed with court office

Forwarding address given to court office

Copy statement obtained

Clinical records needed for trial

Crown Court trial

Court ref		
Patient name		
Date of trial		
Place of trial	Location	Parking
	Accommodation	Train time
Medical records		
Notes		
X-rays		
Copy statement		
Debrief		

Expert witness checklists

Pre-trial

Availability dates sent to solicitor

Letter of terms and conditions sent

Terms agreed

Diary time for preparation

Conference with counsel arranged

All notes available

Witness statements confirmed

Investigation results and methodology available.

Court room skills training arranged

Trial

Date of trial	Location	Parking
Place	Accommodation	Train fare
Documents in bundle		
Notebook		
Report/statement		

6

Personal injury written evidence

Aims

This chapter will help you

- To understand the process of a personal injury case and the healthcare professional's involvement in this process

- To understand the process of preparing reports in personal injury cases

- To produce a template for the writing of such reports

- To analyse the evidence prepared for the other party in the litigation

Introduction

Some people who sustain injuries said to be caused by another individual or corporate body, seek compensation for the injuries themselves and the effect of those injuries.

The patient or client will normally approach a solicitor to act on their behalf. The defendant, be they an individual, or company, is also likely to instruct a legal representative, frequently through their insurer.

Both are likely to instruct healthcare professionals to assist them in the preparation of the case and to provide them with clinical evidence for the court.

In this instance, you are being asked to act as an independent expert witness. Most of these cases begin with a telephone call or letter of instruction from a solicitor, or solicitors from both parties where they are following the personal injury pre-action protocol, or have agreed to co-operate in obtaining the medical evidence or have been ordered to do so by the court.

Experienced solicitors will check by telephone whether your specialist expertise is appropriate for the case especially if you are to be jointly instructed by the other party in the case: both parties may want to know whether and how often you accept instructions from claimants and defendants (**Figure 6.1**).

Dear Sir

Re: **Our client:**..

Address: ....

Date of Accident: ....

We act on behalf of the above mentioned person in connection with an accident. Our client is pursuing a claim for compensation from the person responsible for the accident, and we require a Medical Report in order to prove the claim.

We would be grateful if you could indicate whether you are able to prepare a report on the injuries received by our Client, the treatment given, their present condition and prognosis for recovery.

If you are able to prepare such a report for our purposes, can you please let us know how soon you would be able to see our client, and how quickly a report could be prepared thereafter. Can you please let us know your likely fees.

Our instructions would be offered to you on the basis that you understand that our client is in receipt of Legal Aid and that the amount of fees payable to you will be subject either to authorization or assessment by the Legal Aid Board.

When we receive an indication of your fees, we can make a prompt application to the Legal Aid Board for payment of them and will pass you the payment when received from the Board without delay. Any such payment has to be made on the basis that it does not necessarily reflect the amount that will be allowed on subsequent assessment or taxation, and it is possible, although unlikely, that you could be called upon to make a partial repayment.

We look forward to hearing from you as soon as possible.

Yours faithfully

Figure 6.1 Example of introductory letter

With the withdrawal of legal aid for most personal injury claims from 2000 you will receive variations of this introductory letter in conditional fee and privately paid cases.

What to do on receipt of such a letter

The first thing to do when you receive a letter from a solicitor is to read it thoroughly to ascertain what the solicitor is asking you to do.

The most important part of assessing the letter of instruction is your decision as to whether you are the most appropriate person to prepare this advice or report and whether you are prepared to act on their terms and can do so within the required timetable.

This means that you must have the correct expertise to prepare the report and to give an authoritative opinion on the questions asked about which the lawyer or lawyers requires an opinion. Unless the solicitor has a practice exclusively in personal injury they may be unaware of the differences in the medical specialties such as those between a neurologist and neurosurgeon. In the other healthcare professionals they may not be aware of the difference between the role of a physiotherapist and an occupational therapists role when determining continuing care needs.

The question of fees is covered later in this chapter.

What happens if this initial contact is outside my expertise?

If, on reading the letter, you feel that the area which requires an expert opinion is outside your field of expertise, do not accept the case. If you do, and are subsequently required to attend court, your expertise will be found lacking and a great deal of time and money will be wasted. Your reputation as an expert witness could also suffer.

It is far better to inform the solicitor that, having read the letter, you feel that the request falls outside your expertise and explain to the solicitor exactly where your area of expertise lies.

If you are aware of a someone who is in the appropriate field you could suggest their name to the solicitor. However, by such a recommendation, you may create problems for yourself should the suggested expert not meet the criteria required by the solicitor.

Other questions to ask:

- Is the letter clear as to the specific questions the solicitor(s) need(s) to have answered when applied to this particular case?
- The opinion may be in response to a simple question on a specific injury that the patient has received or it may be asking about the complex rehabilitation needs of a patient who has sustained debilitating injuries.
- If you are instructed by one party only, who is the solicitor representing? (although the report you produce will not depend on the side who instruct you) Some of the practical steps in the preparation of the report may differ depending on the instructing side and it is vital to know the context in which your report is being written.
- Have you previously received instructions from the other side in this particular case? In limited fields this can happen. Generally you will then have a conflict of interest but as the CPR presumption in favour of a single joint expert begins to be adopted you may need to check whether you may now be instructed by both parties.
- What is the time scale given by the solicitor or the court for you to complete the report? Can you meet this deadline? If not you should decline the instructions as the court will rarely extend deadlines for serving or exchanging expert reports merely because the preferred expert is too busy. The party will usually be told to find another expert.
- Have you received the relevant clinical records to prepare the report or has authority been given for you to obtain these records?
- Have you been asked to interview and examine the patient or have you to compile your report purely from written records?

At this stage, it is appropriate to consider whether now is the best time to prepare this report. If the injuries were sustained recently, the present state may not be the final one and a definitive opinion on long term prognosis may not be possible. If you feel this may be an inappropriate time to prepare the report discuss this with the instructing solicitor(s). There may be a legal, rather than clinical, reason for the report at this time e.g a claim cannot be started without a medical report.

Fees and timeframe

Having decided that you are appropriately qualified to prepare the report, and are willing to do so, send an acknowledgment to the instructing solicitors setting out your terms of business (**Figure 6.2**). This must include an estimate of the fee or basis of charging and the terms on which you wish to be paid following invoice submission (this will be covered in detail in Chapter 13). Also, within this letter, inform the solicitor of the time frame you feel will be necessary for you to prepare the report. Request any documents you may require for the report or, where necessary, the authority to obtain these from the person who holds them.

A flexible approach with regard to the timing will allow the solicitor a chance to discuss this with you if they have any questions.

Finally, confirm whether the solicitor wants preliminary advice/report in a letter or as a draft, and if the report is to be prepared as a final document how many top

---

Solicitor's Ref:

Dear Sirs

Your request dated .... to prepare a medical report on under your reference above has been received.

My anticipated fee for providing this report is £225 (based on an hourly rate of £112.50). If attendance at court is required, my daily rate for attending a hearing is £1125. This is equivalent to 10 hours of my hourly rate for preparation and includes travelling and waiting time. Any expenses incurred will be invoiced at cost and copies of receipts for these expenses will be provided.

Payment should be made within 60 days of the date of my invoice.

Please confirm your instructions and I will then send an appointment to your client. I anticipate that the appointment will be .... If a more urgent appointment is required please contact me to discuss this.

I will use my experience, care and skill in fulfilling your instructions to the best of my ability

Yours faithfully

Figure 6.2 Example of acceptance reply

copies of the report the solicitor will require for distribution.

If the solicitor accepts your terms they should confirm their instructions to you including acceptance of your terms or any caveats they may add (**Figure 6.3**).

If you accept these instructions, both parties are bound by the contents of the contract and, as such, have obligations to uphold the conditions of that contract.

Obtaining clinical records

With the introduction of trusts, most hospitals now charge for the photocopying of notes and copying of X-rays. GPs also raise charges. In a complex case records/X-rays may be required by a number of experts. The costs of multiple copies for use by each expert can become expensive. Therefore, many solicitors now obtain the records themselves, copy and bind them and

---

Dear Sir

Re: **Our Client:** ....

   Address: ....

   Telephone No: ....

   Date of Accident: ....

We write further to your letter of 26th November 1996 to confirm that the fees laid down in your letter are acceptable.

We now write to formally request that you prepare a report on the injuries received by our client, the treatment given, present condition and prognosis for recovery. Please contact our client at the address and telephone number set out above to make an appointment to enable you to carry out your examination.

Please remit your fee note and report to ourselves. If there is likely to be a delay in doing so, based upon your original estimate of time to us, can you please keep us informed.

We enclose herewith our client's medical records for your attention.

Yours faithfully

Figure 6.3 Example of confirmation letter

send copies to the expert to help in the preparation of the report. This can also speed up the process.

If, however, the solicitor asks you to obtain the records, it is important that these are sought as early as possible (**Figure 6.4**). For these records to be disclosed to the expert, the request must be accompanied by patient consent (or the parent or legal guardian if the patient is a minor). You should charge for your time in doing this and make this clear to the solicitor.

Which records should I obtain?

Records from hospitals will include medical, nursing and other clinical records and general practitioner records which should be complete showing relevant details prior

---

The Medical Records Office
Nowhere Infirmary
Nowhere

Dear Sir,

re:.............................. DoB ....

I have been requested by the above patient's solicitors to provide a report in connection with a claim for personal injuries sustained on.

The patient attended your hospital as a result of the accident and I would be grateful for a sight of any notes made and X-rays taken with regard to this accident.

I enclose an authorization from the patient to release such information. I confirm that no litigation is contemplated against your hospital or any of your employees.

Any fees incurred in connection with this request should be sent directly to :

Bloggs & Co.
10 High Street
Nowhere

Quoting their ref. ABC/DE/900001

Yours faithfully

Figure 6.4 Example letter to obtain records

to the incident. If there are complex considerations, other records from rehabilitation services may be appropriate.

If you are in doubt about which records you need to see, or are supplied with partial records only, and need to check e.g if the patient/client had any related pre-existing medical condition, you should discuss this with the solicitor(s) who instruct you.

Accident reconstruction and police reports may be helpful in preparing the report, depending on the questions being asked.

The patient's statement may also be helpful but be aware that specific details within the statement may be legally privileged and the solicitor may not wish these details to be disclosed in the report.

Seeing the patient

If the report to be prepared requires an examination of the patient then arrangements must be made for the patient to be seen.

A standard letter should be sent to the patient (**Figures 6.5 and 6.6**), with a copy to the instructing solicitor, giving the date, time and location of the appointment. If you wish to enforce a cancellation fee should the patient fail to attend without prior notice, this should be notified within this letter.

With the introduction by the CPR of much tighter court timetables for production of expert reports than hitherto, especially in Fast Track cases, you will sometimes need to arrange appointments at short notice, or be prepared to decline the instructions. A typical fast track case will reach trial within 30 – 40 weeks of the start of proceedings and you may be asked to prepare a report within 4–8 weeks.

Examination of the patient or investigation of needs

While the format of the examination is similar to assessments made by the healthcare professional during their normal clinical role (and similar standards of care

Dear ....

I have been asked by your solicitor to prepare a report regarding your accident on...............

To prepare this report I require to examine you and have therefore arranged an appointment to see you on .... at .... in .... my Consulting Rooms at the Elsewhere Private Hospital.

If this appointment is not convenient please contact my secretary to arrange an alternative time. **If this appointment is not cancelled a charge of £25 will be levied if you do not attend.**

Yours sincerely

Mr. D. Smith

Consultant in A/E

Figure 6.5 Example appointment letter to client

Dear Sirs

Thank you for your letter confirming your wish for me to prepare a medical report on............................ .

I will be sending an appointment to examine your client in the near future.

I anticipate that this appointment will be on .... at .... in my consulting rooms at ....

If this appointment is not suitable please contact my secretary to arrange an alternative. **If this appointment is not cancelled a charge of £25 will be levied if your client does not attend.**

Yours faithfully

Figure 6.6 Example of copy letter to solicitor

must be exercised in the examination) the result of the investigation must be an independent assessment of the patient's clinical state and his or her needs.

Any investigation should be accompanied by contemporaneous notes. (These are notes made at the time of the investigation or immediately afterwards). This is crucial as these notes may be taken into court and used to refresh the memory. Notes made at a distant time from the event cannot be used and memory alone must be relied on.

If standard investigations are necessary, you may not need to seek prior approval to the additional work/expense. If, however, complex assessments are deemed necessary following an initial examination, it is vital to discuss this with the instructing solicitor(s) before proceeding, particularly as the court now has the power to place a limit on the amount of expert's fees which may be recovered from the losing party to the litigation.

Preparing the report

Many groups have produced a standard format for reports. In this age of technology there is no excuse for unprofessional looking reports (one such style for a medical report is included as Appendix A).

In Summary

- The report must contain information about yourself and your qualifications to produce the report.

- State the purpose of the report, summarise the material instructions (written and oral and/or attach copies of the letters) and state the issues to be addressed within it at the beginning. This may be repeated during the opinion as paragraph headings.

- The relevant historical aspects of the case should be laid out using documentary evidence and the patient's memory.

- Your examination and/or any investigations should be described, together with any further tests, and their results.

- Keep fact and opinion separate.

- Give your opinion and conclusions. If there is a range of professional opinion on an important issue (e.g life expectancy) explain that range, and where your opinion lies within it, with reasons.

- Conclude the report with the declaration that you understand your duty to the court and the statement of truth (that you believe any facts you have started in your report are true) as required by the CPR.

- As appendices, include any supporting material to back up your opinion or to which you have made reference.

- A brief CV should be attached to the report.

What should I do before sending the report?

Prior to submission to the solicitor(s) the report should be read at least twice. The first time to look for obvious errors and the second to check for compliance with instructions, clarity, veracity of your conclusions and consistency in style.

Send the draft (if requested) or prepare the number of top copies you have been asked to provide, sign and date each copy of the report and send them with a fee note to the instructing solicitor.

If you are preparing a joint report you may be asked to send a copy to both sides simultaneously.

Who will see the report?

A report prepared for one party only will initially be seen by the instructing solicitor(s) who will discuss it with their client. When the contents of the report are accepted (see below) the organisation funding the claim, or in larger and more serious claims a barrister or the likely trial advocate may be asked for an opinion as to the case and/or to review the evidence including the report. A medical report on condition and prognosis must be filed at court/served on the defendant when the claim is started.

After the claim has been started, the evidence used to support the case will be given to the other party to the case (i.e. disclosed). This will include the expert report.

At this stage, the report will be seen by the solicitor and the other party, and the advocate and expert advising the other party.

If resolution of the case cannot be reached without a trial, the report will be seen by the judge as part of the evidence presented to the court, by the parties to the action. In legal terms, this evidence forms 'the trial bundle'.

What can happen to the report after it has been initially submitted?

The next stage depends upon the contents of the report and for whom it is written. If the report is prepared on behalf of a claimant, the solicitor will show them the report. The claimant may wish to comment on the contents of the report and the solicitor would then send a copy of these comments to you.

What should you do if asked to modify the report?

Some of the comments may concern the detail of your instructions or be of a factual nature and unless there is evidence from other sources (e.g. written clinical records) that do not support the comments, these amendments can be made. Consequently, if the facts alter this may, in turn, alter the basis for an opinion and therefore, legitimately, the opinion may change.

If, however, the comments are disputing your conclusions, remember your duty is to be an independent witness. If you cannot support the alterations that are being asked, based on the factual evidence including your clinical findings, you should not modify the report, explaining why you believe your conclusions to be correct. At the end of the day, it is the author and signatory of the report who will have to defend its contents in the witness box.

Much has been said about solicitors and their clients attempting to rewrite the reports of experts and to influence the conclusions and the CPR particularly emphasise the role of experts as independent advisors to the court. Judges are trying to stop the partisan expert, but there will be occasions when the courts need to understand the genuinely held opposing views that may occur between practitioners.

In the new world of 'openness' many previously privileged documents are being released, including the letter of instruction to the expert from the solicitor.

CPR 35.10(3) requires experts in reports prepared for use in court proceedings to

"State the substance of all material instructions, written and oral, on the basis of which the report was written"

Moreover Rule 35.10(4) states that (those) instructions "shall not be privileged" and gives the court power to order their disclosure and/or permit questioning in court about them but only when there are "reasonable grounds" to consider the summary in the report to be "inaccurate or incomplete".

This should encourage solicitors to be careful neither to send experts privileged material nor to invite them to write "side letters" on unfavourable aspects of the case nor 'lean' on them to alter unhelpful statements or opinions.

But there are potential problems with this attempted in-road to the well established law of 'privilege' particularly if the courts begin to order disclosure of exchanges of letters with experts when they have been asked to advise about the prospects of a claim at an early stage: it could inhibit a frank exchange of views, or could lead parties and their lawyers to instruct one expert as out of court advisor, and a second expert for court purposes.

What happens when the solicitor sends you the report from the other side for comments?

Sometimes the other side will have expert evidence from another practitioner. When this is disclosed, the instructing solicitor should send you a copy asking for your comments. Remember that the time taken to read the report from the other side, to re-read your notes and report, and prepare a detailed response is chargeable. Ensure that you clear this with the solicitor and send an invoice with comments detailing the time involved.

It is important to deal with the information logically and methodically. When both experts (when there are two) look for the common ground and areas of disagreement, it is then easier for the solicitors to crystallize any area of conflict within the evidence.

How do you reply with comments?

It is important, particularly if some time has elapsed between preparing your report and being asked for comments, to re-read your report. Take note of any investigation or examination that has occurred to the patient and note the date of that examination in relation to your own examination of the patient.

There are two distinct route for comments. Firstly, are the conclusions justified, based on the examination that the other expert carried out? (i.e. if given the same facts would you reach the same conclusions?) Are these facts at variance, even allowing for the passage of time, with the evidence you collected?

If the answer to both questions is yes, the factual basis has possibly changed and you cannot disagree. It may then be appropriate to ask the instructing solicitor if you can re-examine the patient to ascertain whether their clinical status has changed since your initial examination. If, following your examination, you feel that this is so, and the conclusions you draw are now similar to the expert from the other side, then the medical evidence is likely to be agreed and you should state that you agree with the contents of the report.

Secondly, are the conclusions drawn different from the ones you would draw given the similar factual basis? If this applies then there will be a disagreement between the medical experts. In this instance, it is important to be able to provide support for any conclusions you have drawn in your report.

Do not feel intimidated by the status of the expert on the other side, especially if you believe in the opinion you have given and can support it with documentary evidence.

What form should my comments on the other sides report take?

For the sake of clarity, any comments should be written in a report form using both the paragraph numbers in your own report and those of the expert from the other side. Give a point-by-point explanation of the background and your opinion either in support or rebuttal of the conclusions of the other expert.

If the report appears to be lacking in factual information, question this in your response and supply information that you feel justifies your conclusions rather than those of the opposing expert.

Initially, this will be sent to your instructing solicitor, and may possibly be disclosed if the arguments you make are persuasive.

Questions on reports

The CPR have introduced a potentially very helpful new step in procedure – the right to ask questions of an expert in writing within 28 days of receipt of their report (Rule 35.6). The rules do not prescribe a time limit for the expert's reply but 28 days seems a reasonable guideline, unless the court orders otherwise or the trial date is very close.

Experts should be told when their report has been disclosed so they know the timetable for written questions and can plan accordingly. The intention is that 'clarification' questions only will be permitted but it seems likely that parties and lawyers will seek to give this a wide interpretation particularly in Fast Track cases where the expert is unlikely to be giving oral evidence at the trial.

In future, therefore, you may well be asked to help frame questions for the other side's expert. If you have been instructed as a single joint expert by both parties, of course, you may receive two sets of questions.

If the matter still cannot be resolved then any questions you have raised in answer to the other expert's report may be useful to the barrister when preparing his cross-examination of the expert from the other party.

The role of expert meetings and discussions in personal injury

What is an expert meeting?

An expert meeting is a meeting when the experts from both sides consult together in an attempt to resolve any differences. While it has become common practice in other forms of civil litigation, until recently it has not been part of personal injury litigation.

But CPR 35.12 gives the court the power to order experts 'discussions' and these, therefore, are likely to be more frequent in future. In lower value claims and/or where the experts work some distance from one another a telephone discussion will be more "proportionate" than a face-to-face meeting.

Who initiates such a meeting?

The meeting is normally initiated by one of the solicitors although it will usually, in the future, be ordered by the judge in charge of the proceedings. This meeting should be without legal representation and is usually solely with the experts.

As the purpose of the meeting is to settle any disputes between the experts on matters at issue relevant to their opinion evidence, the solicitors should not give instructions as to the precise outcome of the meeting, or on what the experts can or cannot agree, otherwise the meeting serves no purpose except paying lip service to the idea. But the solicitors and experts should agree an agenda in advance.

What constitutes a meeting?

While in the normal sense this would be a face-to-face meeting there is no reason, if the issues appear simple to resolve, that the meeting should not take place by telephone.

How do I prepare for the meeting?

Preparation for this meeting is similar to any forum to discuss the case. It is important that you are familiar with your report and that of the other expert. The legal team may prepare a list of issues and questions to be answered.

You should analyse the areas of agreement and conflict between the reports. Decide whether these are due to differences in the factual basis of the accounts or to differences in interpretation of similar facts.

If your opinion is based on standard works or literature, ensure these are available before and for use during the meeting.

If the meeting is face-to-face dress as appropriate for a professional meeting and arrive in good time at the appointed place. Take a notebook to write down the contents of discussion or, better still, ensure there is a note taker, independent if possible.

What happens at the meeting?

It is important to identify any areas both of agreement and disagreement and these can be written down in a schedule. If there is unanimity of agreement when certain facts are agreed (and remember the expert is not there to decide the facts or legal issues, only give an opinion on the facts) then both experts can agree their conclusions in light of either set of facts.

If, however, there are areas where the opinion on facts is different, it is vital not to agree to anything that you would not feel able to defend in court. During or shortly following this meeting, a joint statement, or answers to questions written and signed by both experts, will be produced and sent to the parties.

Be prepared to listen at the meeting and remain open-minded about the conduct of the case. Do not argue any points just to 'score' over the other expert.

What happens after the meeting?

Following the meeting, or better still, during the meeting, any results are produced as a joint report for both sides in the dispute. This report may be a complete agreement of the expert evidence without qualification, or may be an agreement on the issues should certain facts be accepted. The report may also show some areas may be agreed while others remain unresolved.

If the meeting occurred at an office where facilities are available for immediate dictation, the report should be typed and signed by both experts as a true record of the meeting prior to leaving. Otherwise this report should be produced as soon as possible after the meeting.

The CPR require the note to be placed on the court file although it will only be seen by the trial judge with the parties' consent. The note and any agreement you reach with the other expert will not be 'binding' on the parties but in reality it will be very difficult for a party to set aside or ignore an agreement provided it relates to issues squarely within the expert's domain.

Can the solicitors interfere in the conclusions of such a meeting?

While the solicitors may instruct experts, they should not interfere with what is agreed between two experts at the meeting. Hence some solicitors feel very uncertain about allowing their experts to agree anything at these meetings. Be very clear with your solicitors about what you can and cannot agree.

Checklist for reports

It is important to read the report more than once on completion to ensure that all of the following are present

- A4 good quality paper, hole punched for lever arch file
- Chronology
- Clear headings
- Contents page
- Covering letter and invoice
- Date
- Double spaced or space and a half
- Expressed in the first person
- Front sheet
- Glossary
- Graphics
- Headers on each page
- Margins wide enough for written comments
- Pages and paragraphs numbered
- Publications dated and precede incident date (if appropriate)
- Short sentences and paragraphs
- Signature
- Synopsis

Ensure the report:

- Complies with the requirements of CPR 35.5–10 and the Practice Direction including that it is
- Addressed to the court, not the instructing party(ies)
- Summarises your instructions
- Sets out, where you can, the range of professional opinion on a disputed issue
- Is accurate

- Is concise

- Gives a clear conclusion

- Makes good use of appendices

- Identifies any issues clearly

- Is clear with no jargon that is not explained

- Is logical

- Stands-alone i.e. contains everything that a judge would need

- Clearly cites qualifications and experience

- Contains the required declaration and statement of truth (See Appendix C).

Ask if you would be happy to be cross-examined in court on what you have written?

Remember, the objective is that the report should be EASY for judges and lawyers to use!

Attend a report writing training course to learn more.

7

Personal injury oral evidence

Aims

This chapter will help you

- To understand the process of a civil personal injury case in the courts
- To prepare for a court appearance
- To understand the procedure in a civil court
- To understand cross-examination.

Introduction

Most cases settle without going to court.

What happens if the case cannot be settled?

If there is no agreement by the parties on the evidence, then the matter will be placed for a hearing before a judge in the High or County Court.

An important aim of the civil justice reforms is to provide early trial dates and a clear timetable for service of the evidence to fit in with that date. The court will control the timetable to prevent cases drifting and trials not taking place until years after the accident.

In Fast Track cases, the court will usually fix a two to three week 'trial window' when giving directions when a case is defended. This will be about 30 weeks ahead.

In Multi Track cases, the court may similarly fix a "window" about a year ahead at the case management conference, or in more complex cases delay that step until some evidence has been disclosed.

In both types of case the actual trial date will be fixed later, but at least 8–10 weeks in advance usually after the return of the listing questionnaires.

Solicitors should ask you generally about your availability early in the action before the trial window is arranged and more specifically later before the actual date is fixed, although in Fast Track cases you will very rarely be asked to give oral evidence.

What happens after the trial date is arranged?

Once the date of the hearing has been arranged, the solicitor will contact the expert to notify him or her of the date, time and place of the hearing (**Figure 7.1**). The solicitor is likely to ask for an indication of any fees for attending the hearing including cancellation fees that may be charged, if these have not been agreed at an earlier stage.

Dear Sir

re Bloggs vs Widgets & Co

I write to inform you that the above case in which you have previously prepared a report has been listed for trial at County Court on the 5th and 6th of November 1998.

As the other party has as yet not agreed your evidence it will be necessary for you to attend on these dates to give evidence.

I would be grateful if you will diarise these date and confirm to this office that you are able to attend for both days of the trial.

An indication of your fees for attending the hearing and any terms which apply would be appreciated. Of course any fees would be subject to taxation.

Yours faithfully

Figure 7.1 Example court attendance letter

What do I do?

If the date is fixed and you are able to attend on that date, reply to the solicitor (giving your terms and conditions for attendance (**Figure 7.2**)). If the dispute is about your evidence, then ask for any evidence that you have not seen from the other side (if the report from the expert appointed by the other side has been disclosed and you have commented on it previously, then this may have already crystallised any areas of concern).

How do I prepare for the hearing?

In preparation for the hearing, allocate some time (which is chargeable) before the hearing to review all the evidence you have available. This should include your reports, any ancillary evidence, and any sources including authoritative textbooks. If you have not kept copies of the relevant medical records or you feel there are subsequent records which may be relevant, arrange to see these before the hearing date. A check list for preparing for court is included at the end of this chapter.

Dear Sir

re Bloggs vs Widgets & Co

Thank you for your recent letter indicating the court dates for .... I have reserved both these dates in my diary.

My fees for attending the case are £250 for trial preparation and £1250 per day for attendance at court. This is equivalent to 10 hours of my hourly rate.

The preparation fee will be charged if the case is cancelled within 21 days of the date of the appearance as time will be allocated to the preparation which cannot be reallocated.

If either or both of the days allocated to the case is cancelled within 7 days but before the last working day of the start of the case a fee of 50% of the daily rate will be charged for the day or days so cancelled.

If any day or days not previously cancelled is cancelled within 1 working day of the case commencing the full fee for the time allocated will be charged (although in both instances the preparation fee will be waived).

Yours faithfully

Figure 7.2 Example of reply to solicitor

If you have undertaken investigations, ensure you have both the original results and any subsequent notes available (remember, the hearing may be some time after you prepared the report and your original documents may be filed away).

It is also worthwhile preparing a summary of your qualifications and experience specific to this case. This can be used when introducing yourself to the court as an expert witness. Before attending the court, practice this introduction to ensure that delivery appears confident but not over-confident.

Can I contact the solicitor?

If you are unable to see the area of dispute in the evidence you are presenting, do not hesitate to contact the solicitor. It may be that the solicitor has misinterpreted phrases in the evidence from both sides as being incompatible when they are not.

If there has been a large amount of clinical evidence from a number of specialists a conference with the advocate may be arranged prior to the hearing.

If the case is straightforward, however, the conference is likely to occur in a room within the court building just prior to the hearing. However, if you feel that there is information that the advocate needs to know immediately, contact your instructing solicitor either by telephone or in writing.

Where will the hearing take place?

The hearing will usually take place in a civil trial centre close to the court where the proceedings were started or have been managed. But sometimes hearings may be transferred to another court or trial centre, to even out workloads between courts or to accommodate a witness with special needs.

It is important when preparing for a hearing that the exact location of the building in which the hearing is to take place is known and appropriate travel arrangements including accommodation, if necessary, are made.

What to take to the hearing?

It is important to take with you to court all the relevant notes you have made during your investigation, reports you have submitted and any textbooks or articles you have used in giving your opinion. If there is clinical evidence disclosed from the other side on which you have commented, take that with you plus any references used by the expert appearing on the other side (particularly if you feel that the part of a reference quoted by the expert is taken out of context). Also any questions and answers put to/provided by you and the other expert, and the agreed note of any experts' discussion.

It is also useful to take a duplicate notebook with you as you will be able to sit in court during the evidence and may wish to communicate with the advocate during the examination of other witnesses.

Who should you tell when you arrive in the court building?

It is important to confirm exact arrangements with the instructing solicitor on arrival at court. While the proceedings do not usually commence before 10:30 am, most advocates use the time before the case starts to have a conference with both the factual and expert witnesses. Indeed, in County Court cases, this may be the first time the advocate and the expert witness will have met.

Meetings at the court

Be prepared, during the meeting before the trial commences, for the advocate to ask searching questions. He is not doubting your expertise or experience but testing the evidence just as the opposing advocate is likely to do when you are in the witness box.

At this stage, the strengths and weaknesses in the evidence should be pointed out to the advocate and solicitor. This is not partisanship by the expert but it is important to give a balanced and impartial opinion based on the evidence. If a question is asked which you feel requires a negative answer then tell the advocate and solicitor.

Sometimes in the weeks immediately prior to the court hearing, both sides attempt to settle on a figure for compensation. The expert may be asked to advise especially on matters which affect the likely compensation e.g the ability of the client to work at a specific job, or if all work will now be difficult, or the exact care needs of the client.

Conduct of the case

Many cases settle during the last few days before the hearing commences, some even on the day of the trial, although the CPR rules on offers to settle should lead to fewer last minute settlements, which can be very stressful for the lay client.

In addition, there may be agreement reached on the evidence during the pre-trial phase. A meeting of the expert witnesses to narrow the areas of disagreement may be arranged, or even ordered, by the judge.

The conduct of such meetings, which are common in commercial litigation but less so in medical litigation, is covered in the previous chapter.

The court

In a civil case the matter is decided by a judge sitting on his/her own. Usually the evidence is presented first by the claimant and then by the defence. Normally, witnesses of fact are called prior to witnesses of opinion (the expert witnesses).

However, as the expert witnesses can only give opinions based on the facts they are often asked to sit in court during the proceedings. They sit behind the advocate presenting the case for the party who has instructed them. Should a fact come to light during the hearing that causes an expert to change the opinion given in their report they should communicate that fact to the advocate.

Often, during the case, the advocate may ask the expert witnesses for clarification of a point being made by a witness of fact and this may influence the line of questioning that occurs. It is therefore important to listen to the evidence, particularly if it is different from the evidence given in statements the expert witness has seen prior to the court hearings.

Giving evidence

When giving evidence there are rules of procedure that must be adhered to. Any item taken into the witness box may be examined by the opposing advocate. It is therefore better not to take a copy of any report you have made into the witness box which contain hand-written notes. It is better to rely on the copy of the report which has been prepared for the court and presented in evidence prior to the hearing (which will be in the court bundle).

Do not take any other textbooks or even electronic copies of the report into the witness box as the contents of the entire computer organiser system may be examined by the advocate. This is especially important if an undisclosed letter has been written to the solicitor and a copy of this letter is on the hard disk of the computer.

Taking the oath

On entering the witness box, the expert witness will be asked to take the oath or to affirm. The holy book on which you wish to take the oath should be communicated to the court usher before entering the witness box.

Establishing your right to act as an expert

While there is no legal definition of an expert witness, the criterion for accepting evidence from a person in the role of an expert depends upon them establishing to the court that they have qualifications and expertise in the field of dispute. It is also important that the knowledge and expertise must be relevant to the time the incident occurred. Normally, the advocate will ask the expert witness to give their name, qualifications and current appointment. The expert then gives an account of their experience with particular reference to the specific case being heard and the evidence in dispute.

Examination in chief

After establishing the expertise of the expert, the advocate will turn to the evidence in chief. In order to streamline proceedings, many courts accept the report as the evidence in chief. This questioning may be limited to asking if your report is your opinion based on the facts as you were aware of them at the time, and if anything you have heard in the court has altered your opinion as presented in your report.

Cross-examination

After this, the advocate for the other party to the proceedings will ask you questions. Remember that if he is presenting any expert evidence he will have an expert sitting behind him listening to your evidence and who may be giving him advice during your evidence.

Cross-examination has two major elements. The questioning of evidence you are giving and questioning your expertise to give the evidence you have presented.

This cross-examination may include techniques developed to unsettle the witness (e.g appearing disinterested or interrupting or trying to needle the witness). Remember that these tactics are deliberate and do not become annoyed at the advocate.

The advocate from the other side may ask you to compare yourself with the expert appearing on his side in an unfavourable light.

He may also ask about any investigations that you carried out whilst preparing your report. Remember if he asks about a test you have not heard of, request an explanation or ask to be given time to consider the background evidence which demonstrates the relevance of the test.

The advocate may ask you about the facts of the case in the light of the factual evidence presented to the court. However, if you have changed your view about the opinion based on the factual evidence this should have been communicated to the advocate before you even entered the witness box.

Finally, the advocate may imply that the evidence you are giving is biased because you represent one side or the other and, as such, your evidence should be disregarded. If you have prepared your evidence in a balanced way then this accusation is groundless.

If you want to experience cross-examination in a training environment before being exposed to it in court, there are training courses which cover this (see **Appendix D**).

Re-examination

Following cross-examination, the advocate for the party who called you may re-examine you if there were points raised in cross-examination that require clarification. He cannot raise new issues at this stage.

Answering questions

No matter how simple a question seems or how stupid it may appear, virtually all questions should be answered thoughtfully in a calm and measured way. If at all possible, the contents of the report should be used to explain each opinion, and the reference in the report should be pointed out to the advocate in a courteous manner.

While every profession has their own 'shorthand' it is best to avoid use of this while in the witness box. Explain the contents of the report in language easily understood by a lay person. If it is impossible to avoid using a technical term because a lay explanation is not precise, give the technical term followed by the nearest equivalent in lay terms.

If you are describing injuries or mechanisms of injury, remember that your own body may be used as an anatomical model as a means of explanation to the judge.

Whom should I address?

All the answers to questions should be directed at the judge hearing the case. Every question should be seen as an opportunity to explain to the judge the core of the evidence presented. Answers should also address any weaknesses in the case ensuring these have been considered and that a balanced view has been taken.

8

Conferences with the advocates

Aims

This chapter will demonstrate

- The format of a conference

- How to prepare for a conference

- The conduct of a conference

- How the results of a conference may influence further proceedings

Introduction

What is a conference with an advocate?

A conference with an advocate is the legal term for a meeting between a barrister and/or a solicitor advocate instructed to give advice on a case with the party whom they represent.

A healthcare professional may attend these meetings:

- as a defendant in a case of clinical negligence;

- as a witness to fact in a professional role in a criminal case;

- as an expert witness to aid the conduct of the case.

Where does a conference take place?

The conference may take place in the chambers of the barrister or a mutually convenient place for all parties. It may also take place as a conference call by telephone between the barrister/advocate and an expert.

However, in simple criminal and personal injury cases, the conference may take place at the court on the day of the hearing. These conferences are discussed in Chapter 4.

When does a conference take place?

Many conferences take place in the late afternoon following the day's court work. If the issues to be dealt with are complex, they may not finish until very late.

Sometimes, the conference may occur some months after the original report has been prepared and it may be necessary to have a series of conferences necessary as the litigation proceeds through its various stages.

How do I prepare for a conference?

After a report has been prepared, the solicitor will usually telephone or write asking the healthcare professional for possible dates on which to hold a conference (**Figure 8.1**).

Dear Sir

re Bloggs vs Southern NHS Trust

We write further to your reports on the above case.

All the evidence in the case has been reviewed by counsel and we now wish to arrange a conference with all the experts.

Counsel is available during the weeks commencing 4th & 11th November and I would be grateful for any days during that period which you are unable to attend at 4:30 pm in London.

A note of your fees for attendance for the conference would also be appreciated.

Yours faithfully

Figure 8.1 Letter arranging conference

You must be prepared for this at any time after you have prepared a report and should identify a range of possible dates for the solicitor and your terms for attending the conference (**Figure 8.2**).

Dear Sirs

re Bloggs vs Southern NHS Trust

Thank you for your letter regarding dates for a conference on the above case. Any evening apart from Wednesday 5th November is suitable for me and I await confirmation of the exact date.

My fees for attending the conference are £125 per hour for the period of the conference and £62.50 for the travelling time by train which would be approximately 2 hours in each direction. In addition expenses, including a first class train fare, would be chargeable.

I would appreciate at least 7 days notice to re-arrange any other commitments and if there are any changes to my availability prior to confirmation of a date I will inform you immediately.

Yours faithfully

Figure 8.2 Reply letter

The solicitor will ordinarily have a number of people, all of whom have to attend the conference including the lay client and other experts. He or she will try to accommodate all of these parties. If you state that you are able to attend on a specific day and the solicitor arranges a conference for that day and time it is your professional duty to be available i.e. once you have given provisional dates you should not book anything else for that time until the solicitor has confirmed an alternative date).

Confirmation of conference

The solicitor will then write to you confirming the final details of the conference, the date, time and place and agreement of your fees for attendance.

If the conference takes place outside your area then a map or directions should be enclosed with this letter.

Preparing for the conference

The preparation for a conference is similar to that for a court appearance. You should review all relevant case records, including your report and any other reports given to you for comment.

You should prepare all the supporting documentation used in preparation of your report and take copies of any papers or parts of textbooks referred to within your and any other relevant report.

Annotate anything you feel supports your opinion in the records so that you can refer to it easily in the collection of papers during the conference. Do not forget to take a notebook and pen.

Getting to the conference

Make sure that you will arrive at the conference on time. If you have a long journey then some of the final preparation can be done en route to the conference if travelling by train. Know where you are going and add extra time for travel in case there are any delays.

Take all the relevant papers with you as you cannot rely on a set being available at the conference.

The conduct of the conference

The conference is normally chaired by the advocate but may be introduced initially by the instructing solicitor who will probably know all the parties concerned.

The conduct of the conference will depend both on the advocate and the issues to be discussed. Expect that during the conference your evidence will be tested and your opinion questioned, particularly if there is evidence from the other side that results in a different conclusion from that stated in your evidence.

While the healthcare professional may feel aggrieved that their word is being questioned the purpose of this questioning is twofold.

- Firstly, this approach will test the evidence itself and ensure that it will stand up if presented to court.

- Secondly, it will show whether, under questioning, the healthcare professional can stand by their report and justify their actions or the opinion they have given. The advocate is making a professional judgement as to the quality of the healthcare professional as a witness.

Technical discussions may also take place in the conference particularly if there are a large number of healthcare professionals involved in the various aspects of the case.

Each may have prepared a report independently and there may be areas of overlap or potential conflict in the evidence. At the conference these will be aired and a conclusion reached as to how these issues are to be resolved.

During the conference a member of the legal team will keep a note of the proceedings but should anything important arise for your action following the conference, it is vital to take your own notes of these events.

Do not be intimidated at the conference: if your opinion was not valued, your evidence would have been discarded long before the conference.

Remember that the report you have written is your work and if used in evidence must be signed and presented to court under your name. Do not feel that you have to please the legal team by agreeing with changes to the report. At the same time, if the phraseology of your original report appears unclear, a form of words to clarify your position may be suggested. The changes to the report will clarify that opinion.

9

Medical negligence defendant

Aims

This chapter will help

- The health care professional to understand the procedures involved in defending a medical negligence case

- To advise the healthcare professional on the steps to take if they are involved in such a case

- Explain in outline the clinical negligence preaction protocol

Introduction

One of the most worrying letters a healthcare professional can receive is one which alleges that they have committed a negligent act (**Figure 9.1**). This normally comes in a solicitor's letter asking for access to the health records of a patient under the Access to Health Records Act or Data Protection Act.

Dear Mr Bloggs

re: Mr Claim

I am acting for the St Elsewhere NHS Trust with regard to a possible claim against the trust by the above patient.

The claim is in respect of a period of treatment that the patient underwent in the above hospital during the period January to June 1997. The solicitors for the patient are alleging that there was a failure to properly investigate Mr Claim when he first attended the hospital in January 1997 and as a result the correct diagnosis was delayed for a period of 9 months. A referral to a private practitioner resulted in the need for additional treatment to relieve his problems.

I enclose herewith a copy of the letter from the solicitor dated 1 April 1999 giving more details of the allegations and copies of the medical records from St Elsewhere Hospital. There are also copies of letters from the private consultant to whom Mr Claim was subsequently referred, detailing the diagnosis and treatment he performed. The initial records have already been disclosed to the plaintiff's solicitor.

As you were one of the doctors who was involved with the care of Mr Claim during the period when the alleged negligence occurred I would be grateful if you could prepare a report dealing with the treatment you gave to Mr Claim during the relevant period and commenting on the specific allegations in the solicitor's letter.

Your initial comments will of course only be seen by myself and any expert instructed by this firm to independently review the care that Mr Claim received.

If in due course the claim proceeds, this report will be prepared in a form to be presented as evidence to the court.

Many thanks for your assistance and I look forward to hearing from you.

If you require any further information please do not hesitate to let me know.

Yours faithfully

Figure 9.1 Example of initial letter regarding a claim

Most of these letters are directed to the administrative section of the hospital and these are passed on to their legal advisors.

The CPR introduced the use of a clinical negligence pre-action protocol (see Annex) which requires the potential claimant to send a full letter of claim to the healthcare body at least three months before issuing proceedings. The intention is to give the organisation time to investigate and to respond, at least to the allegations of negligence, so that if liability is accepted the parties can continue to exchange information relevant to the value of the claim and try to settle it without litigation. If the organisation does not admit liability, a reasoned letter of response is required and copies of relevant documents including medical records should be sent to the patient's solicitor then, if they have not previously been requested. In complex or difficult cases the three month period might be extended by negotiation. Full letters of claim adopting the protocol approach should always be taken seriously and the case carefully investigated.

In an attempt to reduce costs, many of the simple administrative tasks involved in preparing the case to defend a medical negligence claim are performed by employees of the healthcare organisation involved. They often ask for initial statements from the senior personnel involved before passing the case to the legal advisors for an overview. If there is sufficient evidence that the case is likely to be pursued, the healthcare organisation then starts to obtain evidence from the personnel involved.

As there is often a delay between the alleged action of negligence and the initiation of a claim, many of the personnel involved in the alleged claim may have left the organisation and therefore have to be contacted by a letter.

What to do in these circumstances?

Firstly, do not panic. Secondly, gather support to answer the allegation.

If the problem arose in an NHS hospital most of the indemnity is covered under their scheme, including the CNST. Alternatively, if the problem arose in the private sector, the first port of call for you is your professional indemnity insurance scheme.

Establish your involvement in the case, particularly in relation to the allegations. Sometimes this may result in searching through many clinical records looking for your signature. Once you have identified that you were involved with the care of the patient, review the notes you made at the time.

Ask yourself if you remember the patient but bear in mind that contact may have been some years ago. Look again at the allegation made in the claim because usually the health trusts's legal department will ask for statements from involved individuals before an official statement of claim is made. The legal department may have received a request for the medical records merely suggesting a potential claim.

Preparing the factual statement

Having looked at the notes, the next stage is to give a factual statement regarding your involvement in the patient's care.

The introduction should include your name, professional qualifications now and at the time of the incident. Your current employment should also be recorded if it is different from that at the time of the incident.

The actual appointment held at the time of the incident should be recorded followed by a narrative account of what occurred. Hopefully, this will be fully documented in the clinical records. If there are factual omissions which you remember, these can be included in the statement. However, you should note the reason for recalling these items and why they were not recorded in the original notes.

Having completed the factual part of the statement, a summary of your initial response to the allegations can be made. In this part of your statement, you should make reference to your normal practice in the circumstances you found at the incident. You should justify reasons for this practice.

If the allegations pertain to an area where you have published work in the public domain, then both the reference and a copy of the relevant paper should be added to your statement before submitting it to the legal team acting on your behalf.

Should you ask for advice before sending the statements?

The legal advisors to the health care organisation are acting on its behalf and although they will also be representing the individual professional, they are employed to give advice to the organisation *not* to the individual.

If there are specific allegations against you as an individual which may lead to a conflict between your reputation as an individual and the corporate responsibility of the legal advisors to the trust then you should seek independent advise about the contents of your statement from a professional indemnity organisation before it is submitted to the health care organisation's legal advisors.

What happens next?

If your involvement was peripheral to the specific allegations (e.g. you gave the patient an uneventful anaesthetic during a long hospital admission) then having completed and submitted your statement there may be no more involvement for you in the case.

If, however, your actions are central to the allegations of sub-standard care, the next stage in the proceedings will usually be to convert your statement, which is a privileged document, into a witness statement. This will be disclosed and added to the bundle seen by the expert employed to give independent advice to the legal team.

You should be ready to answer in detail any questions regarding action or lack of action undertaken by you. Do not take offence at this as the legal advisor is simply testing your evidence as will be done if the case ever comes to court. It is far better for the difficult questions to be asked early, a view on liability taken, and early settlement of a legitimate claim made rather than dragging out the process. Similar questions may come up in open court with the press reporting every word, exposing you to unwanted scrutiny and possible loss of reputation.

Following completion of the witness statement there may be some delay before anything happens. During this time the legal team will be obtaining expert clinical evidence from independent expert witnesses to help them decide if there is a reasonable chance of defending the case or whether settlement should be explored.

If you move jobs, remember to inform someone involved in the case and supply a new contact address.

Do not assume that the case has been settled or abandoned if you hear nothing for some time.

If the case does not settle or if there are issues to be clarified, a meeting of the entire team involving both the professional witnesses of fact, the expert witnesses and the legal team may take place. The conduct of this meeting is discussed in Chapter 8.

If a settlement seems possible you may be asked to attend a negotiating meeting or mediation particularly if the patient/claimant wants a face-to-face discussion with you.

10

Medical negligence liability: written evidence

Aims

This chapter will

- Give an outline of the procedures in clinical negligence

- Show how an appropriate report is commissioned on liability

- Give an outline of the preparation of such a report

- Give advice regarding the final report for disclosure

- Help you to respond to written evidence from the other party

Introduction

In order for a claimant to prove that a healthcare professional was negligent in giving the plaintiff treatment they have to show that:

- there was a duty of care;

- there was a breach of that duty;

- the breach of duty resulted in damage; and

- the damage was a direct result of the breach of duty.

To establish each of these, there is a need for expert evidence and the defendant health authority or individual practitioner (normally through their professional indemnity insurer) will also have expert witnesses.

Often the experts used to establish each of these parts of the negligence claim are from differing specialist areas and it is important that, as a healthcare professional involved in this work, this is appreciated.

The injury the plaintiff has suffered may be similar to the injuries sustained in accidents where the negligence is from another source (i.e. road traffic accident) and the type of condition and prognosis report produced in this instance is similar to that produced for personal injury claims.

However, the report which establishes the breach of duty (i.e. the liability report), is completely different. A healthcare professional must have some knowledge of the legal background that this involves.

The expert chosen to give an opinion on liability in these cases must work in the same discipline and area of expertise as the healthcare professional against whom the allegation is made.

It is also important that the expert has knowledge of the work environment of the alleged allegation. For instance, if a patient has suffered brain damage as a result of an accident and it is alleged that the hospital where they were first admitted did not treat them properly, the expert chosen to prepare a report should be from the same discipline as that of the admitting hospital's head injury team and should work in a similar type of establishment and have done so at the date of the treatment in question.

Similarly, if the allegation is against a physiotherapist in private practice, the report should be submitted by a practitioner in a similar field.

The initial letter

Most requests to undertake a liability report commence with a telephone call or letter from a solicitor asking if you are prepared to act and including brief details about the case (**Figure 10.1**).

Dear Sir

I have been instructed by Miss Smith to pursue a claim against the War Memorial NHS trust for alleged clinical negligence and you have been recommended to give an expert opinion.

In brief, my client instructs me that she attended the War Memorial Hospital on several occasions over a period of weeks having on occasions attended herself and on other occasions being referred by her GP to various specialists. On each occasion she was discharged home until on the last she was admitted complaining of abdominal pain and severe vomiting.

She complained that she was not admitted previously, nor were appropriate investigations carried out and as a result she had to be admitted as an emergency case for surgery to be carried out.

I confirm that I have in my possession the complete hospital records and General Practitioner records of my client and these have been ordered and paginated.

Before we can instruct you formally we need to know what your fee would be so that we can seek specific authority from the Legal Aid Board.

In addition to an estimate of your fees and your time scale for preparing the report we would be grateful if you would confirm that there is no conflict of interest in dealing this matter and that you have not previously been instructed to prepare expert evidence in this case on behalf of any other party.

Once we have received specific authority from the Legal Aid Board we can formally instruct you and forward the medical records to you.

Yours faithfully

Figure 10.1 Example letter of approach

What happens next?

Having received your letter the solicitor will normally apply to the Legal Aid Board client or funder of the claim for approval for the report (see Chapter 13)

If the Legal Aid Board accepts your terms and the solicitor wishes to instruct you they will send a formal letter of instruction (**Figure 10.3**).

This will usually include a more detailed account of the allegations being made and often some indication of the exact questions the solicitor wishes you to answer.

At this point, the solicitor will enclose the clinical records of the patient, together with statements from witnesses of fact that have been obtained.

The solicitor will normally also give you some of the legal background to the burden of proof in clinical negligence.

Having received this letter there are some immediate actions that you should undertake to smooth the subsequent management of the case.

Take a brief look at all the notes to ensure that the solicitor has provided all the relevant papers to allow you to prepare the report. Having seen the extent of the clinical and other material, is the time you estimated for preparation of the report correct?

Bear in mind that a detailed look at the contents of these records will not occur until the actual report is prepared. This will take place according to the timetable you set down in the terms you sent to the solicitor. If any records or other material appear to be missing, inform the solicitor immediately.

If the quantity of material is much greater than you were led to believe in the initial letter and you feel that the estimate you gave to the solicitor originally was too low, write to the solicitor explaining why and send a revised estimate including the reasons for the change. Before commencing any work on the report, you must wait for the solicitor to agree to this revision.

At this stage, if all the records are present and the estimate you gave is approximately correct, it is important to prepare a diary note indicating the

Dear Sir

Further to previous correspondence I am pleased to confirm that I now have authority from the Legal Aid Board to incur your fee to a maximum of £750. If your fee is likely to exceed this sum we should be grateful if you would come back to us prior to preparing your report so that we may obtain revised authority from the Legal Aid Board.

We now attach: -

1.   Records from the hospital
2.   GP records
3.   My client's initial statement
4.   Our client's comments in relation to the medical records

My client instructs me that she attended the War Memorial Hospital on several occasions over a period of weeks having on occasions attended herself and on other occasions being referred by her GP to various specialists. On each occasion she was discharged home until on the last she was admitted complaining of abdominal pain and severe vomiting.

She complained that she was not admitted previously nor were appropriate investigations carried out and as a result she had to be admitted as an emergency case for surgery to be carried out.

My client also alleges that the scarring with which she has been left is not acceptable and that this either resulted from the way in which the surgery was performed or alternatively the fact that surgery was necessary as a matter of emergency.

I should be grateful if you would consider the standard of treatment received by my client and whether this fell below the reasonably expected standard of care. If you do believe the treatment received fell below the reasonably expected standard of care I should be grateful if you could consider what avoidable damage and harm has been suffered by my client as a result of any negligence. I am asking the other expert instructed Dr_____to deal with the question of condition and prognosis so should be grateful if you could consider the issues of liability in relation to the treatment at the Accident & Emergency department.

In view of the fact that she had a large cyst and appendicitis I presume that she would have needed surgery in any event. I should be grateful if you would consider whether she should have been admitted on her first attendance at casualty and whether this would have made any difference to the treatment later offered. Would she still have required surgery as a matter of urgency?

I am asking another expert, Mr_____, to consider the way in which the surgery was actually performed as my client is concerned at the resulting scarring.

The test that my client has to satisfy in order to succeed in a claim against the health authority is that the standard of care received by her fell below that standard that should have reasonably been expected from a body of medical practitioners at the time treatment was given in January 1993.

It would be very helpful if you could support your report with reference to standard leading textbooks, publications etc. and where possible provide photocopies or extracts of these.

I look forward to receiving your report in due course and thank you for your help in this matter.

Yours faithfully

Figure 10.3 Formal letter of instruction

timetable to prepare the report (ensuring that you keep to the schedule agreed in your terms).

Preparing the report

There are three parts to a liability report.

- what happened (the historical narrative)
- what should have happened (the expected standard of care)
- what went wrong (the breach of those standards)

While every expert has their own layout of reports the above outline shows one method of dividing opinion from facts. It demonstrates to the solicitor, and others who subsequently see the report, the clarity of your thinking.

Reading the factual documents

The factual documents may include not only copious clinical records but statements from witnesses of fact from the party who has instructed you.

There may also be some correspondence from the defendant trust if the patient has followed the complaints procedure or you are being instructed after the clinical disputes preaction protocol has been followed.

Finally, if there has been a death and an inquest has been convened, witness statements used in that forum may be available.

Clinical records

When reading the clinical records try not to look at them with the benefit of hindsight. When the diagnosis or treatment is clear, many things may appear to fall below the acceptable level of care. However, the healthcare professional works within an area where there is often no exact right or wrong, and information may be incomplete at the commencement of contact between the patient and the healthcare worker.

It is important for the expert witness reading the records to put themselves in the place of the healthcare professional receiving the information as documented in the records. The expert witness should view the subsequent actions of the healthcare professional in the light of the information that was obtained at the time.

It should be appreciated that the information in the notes may be at conflict with the evidence of the witness statements in the case, particularly that of the claimant. When reading the clinical records and the witness statements it is advisable to maintain a healthy scepticism for the accuracy these records and statements.

Read the records and the statements from the witnesses noting any similarities or differences between them and the written records.

Writing the narrative

The narrative section of the report can be written once all documents have been read. If there are two different accounts of the circumstances, record both of these in the report as alternative explanations, without at this stage commenting on the differences.

If there are reports from other experts which tell the narrative particularly about an area outside your own field, give a brief summary of this part of the circumstances as you will not be asked for an opinion regarding that part of the case.

Defining the standard of care

Having read and recorded the narrative section of the report, the next logical step is to define the acceptable standard of care for any patient presenting to a healthcare professional of equal grade at that particular time with the same problem.

Within this, there may be a variety of similar standards which could be adopted, according to the interpretation of various factors, in the history and initial assessment of the patient. Any relevant texts current at the time of the incident should be consulted for an authoritative view of acceptable standards of care. Sometimes, the relevant guidelines produced by statutory bodies may be helpful.

Writing the opinion

The opinion is often the most difficult part of a report to write. Firstly the facts may be in dispute, i.e. the patient and the healthcare professional may have different perceptions of the consultation between them. Remember that it is not for the expert witness to define the facts of the case but only to define whether the standard of care was acceptable.

If there are two differing accounts, then an opinion must be given for each set of facts. In the report, the expert witness must remain objective. If there was an acceptable standard of care in some parts of the treatment but not in others it is necessary for the expert to acknowledge this. It should be stated the expert witness feels that some of the allegations have not been substantiated. However, the expert witness may find that the overall standard of care was below an acceptable level.

Deal with each part of the case logically and in sequence as often the series of events that occur are additive and it is the total 'package' of care the patient received that was unacceptable.

Writing the conclusions

Having written the whole report the expert should compile a summary of the main facts, including his opinion. This should be brief and placed at the beginning of the report.

Appendices

Any literature used to help form the opinion should be copied and appended to the report. In addition to the relevant section, the title page and publication details should also be supplied as information for the legal team and, after exchange, to allow the expert on the other side to see your literature review.

A single page CV should be appended to the report.

Who will see this initial report?

The initial report will be seen by the solicitor and the client only, if proceedings have not been started. Following this, there may be questions raised about the report by the solicitor and if the report is favourable on liability the solicitor may proceed to obtain other reports on causation and the injuries themselves, from other healthcare professionals.

What happens next?

If favourable, the report will be used to prepare a protocol letter of claim and/or together with the witness statements, will be used by the solicitor or possibly counsel to produce a statement of case. This will convert into legal wording the opinion of the expert in relationship to the care received by the patient.

Usually, you will be asked for your opinion on this document before it is submitted to the other side. If you feel that the document does not truly represent your view, the solicitor should be told which of the points does not accord with your opinion and why. It may be that the statement is based on the witness statements that accord with the case being pursued and may not, therefore, be as impartial as the opinion given in your report.

The report for disclosure

After proceedings have been started/defended and the witness statements have been exchanged, the solicitor will normally send all the documentation to the expert witness to ask if the documents or witness evidence enclosed alter or change his or her opinion. It may be that, in light of these documents, the expert witness changes their view on the standard of care, or an alternative set of facts is presented that the expert is unable to confirm as the truth and may simply reinforce the opinion given on each set of facts.

At this stage the solicitor will probably ask the expert to prepare his or her final report for disclosure, incorporating any new evidence or the results of discussions that have taken place between the legal and clinical teams (see Chapter 8).

Having prepared this report, (and in accordance with the CPR and any specific court requirements) it should be signed and sent to the solicitor with the number of copies the solicitor has requested.

Reading other reports

What happens if another expert acting on the same side argues with my conclusions?

Sometimes, despite the solicitor asking specific experts to act within their own field, some try to express opinions outside that field of expertise and they may undermine another specialist. One expert may identify a point that another expert has missed. If this is the case the expert should consider the inclusion of any such points within their report.

If, however, the expert is trying to give an expert view on the clinical care given by another profession or speciality then it is the responsibility of the expert to robustly defend their corner.

This often happens in newly emerging specialities when more established practitioners feel they know best how the care of patients in that area should be undertaken. While healthcare practitioners in more established specialities may have *some* knowledge if they do not work within that area, they are not deemed to be expert in that area.

What happens when the expert report on the other side is disclosed?

The final piece of evidence an expert on liability has to consider is the report from the expert on the other side.

If that expert has produced a report based on all the relevant facts, it may be similar to your report giving the opinion based on two differing accounts. If this is the case, and the conclusions drawn are the same as yours (apart from the varying facts) then the judge will decide the facts and the opinion on liability will be the same from both experts (if the case does not settle).

If the expert presents some facts that you did not find, either in the notes or the documents, you must examine these and, if they change your opinion, it is your duty to advise your instructing solicitor of this.

If there is evidence from either a publication or textbook that you have not considered, then identify this and assess it with regard to your report. Again, if this forms an acceptable standard of care, then it is your duty to report this to your instructing solicitor.

Remember to clear with the solicitor the fees for the time you will take to review the other expert's report.

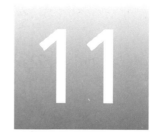

11

Medical negligence: oral evidence

Aims

This chapter will

- Show the procedures followed when preparing for a medical negligence trial

- Help prepare the healthcare professional for the trial

- Aid understanding of the mechanics of the trial

- Show how the procedure of the trial will unfold

- Help the healthcare professional in giving evidence at a medical negligence trial

Introduction

If a case of clinical negligence cannot be settled by an offer to settle payment into court, negotiation or ADR, a trial will take place.

There are three areas where potential disagreement can occur. The trial may concentrate on one or more areas. These are:

- liability;

- causation;

- the injury suffered.

Before the trial commences there may be agreement between the parties on any of these issues and the expert evidence on those issues will not then be in dispute.

What starts the trial process?

Most clinical negligence cases will be allocated by the court to The Multi Track. The case managing judge will 'fix a trial window' or date when giving directions and/or at a case management conference. You are likely to be asked about your availability within the 'window' some months in advance. A definite date will be fixed at least several weeks, and often longer in advance.

Having given availability for a specific time, do not make other commitments for that time without first contacting the solicitor.

When approached for prospective dates, the solicitor will invariably request terms for attending court. If this is more than a year ahead then remember that your fees may increase during the interim period and this should be included in the assessment (see **Figure 11.1**).

The solicitor will, having arranged a court date, inform the expert witness of the dates set aside for the trial and whether attendance will be necessary for the entire period. Often, the fixing of a trial date encourages discussions about settlement, and a flurry of correspondence requiring attention ensues.

Smith & Jones
Solicitors
New Court Road
Harrow

Dear Sirs

re Mr Bloggs

Thank you for your recent letter indicating the court dates for .... I have reserved these dates in my diary.

My fees for attending the case are £250 for trial preparation and £1000 per day for attendance at court. This is equivalent to 10 hours at my hourly rate.

The preparation fee will be charged if the case is cancelled within 21 days of the date of the appearance as time will be allocated to preparation which cannot be reallocated.

If any day allocated to the case is cancelled within 7 days but before the last working day of the start of the case a fee of 50% of the daily rate will be charged for the day or days so cancelled.

If any day or days not previously cancelled is cancelled within 1 working day of the case commencing the full fee for the time allocated will be charged (although in both instances the preparation fee will be waived).

Any fees incurred will be billed at the conclusion of the court appearance and will be due for payment within 60 days of invoice.

I would appreciate your written confirmation of these terms

Yours faithfully

Figure 11.1 Example of Terms of Agreement Letter

At this stage, depending on the outcome of the correspondence and if the area of dispute is small, the need to go to trial and give evidence may be avoided.

As in personal injury claims, parties will have the opportunity to put written questions to experts on their reports, and the court may order, or the parties may themselves arrange, a discussion or meeting between experts of the same discipline.

Preparing for trial

There are two aspects to cover in preparation for trial, particularly if it is a large case being tried in a centre far away from the home base: preparation of the evidence and logistic preparation.

Preparing the evidence

Many clinical negligence cases last a significant time from start to finish. The initial report and the report disclosed to the other party may have been prepared some years before the trial date. Therefore, before the trial, all reports should be reviewed, together with any questions and answers, and notes of experts' meetings, and any further notes, together with the relevant pages of the clinical records should be checked. This is vital as during the trial the advocate will be referring to the expert for advice on both the factual and expert evidence within their field.

Look both at the strengths and weaknesses in the evidence and prepare a summary of your evidence and opinion both for your own benefit and for discussion with the legal team.

It is important in the preparation for trial that the expert gives due consideration to the area of his own expertise and experience and prepares an appropriate aide memoire to help present this expertise. This will be useful to refer to when the advocate seeks to establish the credibility of the expert witness.

Time spent in preparation is chargeable and may either be included in the charge for the court appearance or invoiced for separately.

Contact with the legal team

Informal contact may have taken place with the legal team prior to the trial to answer any points contained within the evidence. A pre-trial conference may also be arranged. The advocates and all the witnesses may attend this before the trial.

Arrangements for such a meeting are the same as those for any other conferences with counsel. However, there is a sense of urgency because of the deadline of a trial date.

Logistic preparation

When the date, place and length of the trial are known a decision should be made whether to travel there and back each day or to travel the night before and stay in a hotel. Decide on both the method and the timing of the journey.

If bookings need to be made, agreement should be obtained for reimbursement of any expenses incurred.

In addition to any general travel arrangements, the site of the court and availability of local parking should be checked.

The day before the trial

The day before the hearing is the time to collect all the material to take to court. In addition to both your annotated copy of the clinical records and report you should take the complete textbooks and papers you have used in the preparation of the report or reports. This can often include a great deal of papers and may influence your decision about travel.

If the trial is anticipated to last a few days and accommodation has been arranged away from home, adequate clothing should be taken.

Should access be needed to technology (computers, pagers etc.) then arrange this. When in the court environs, however, the use of mobile phones and pagers is discouraged.

If you have not arranged for time away from your employment and need to be contacted, remember to leave contact numbers with all those who need to know your whereabouts.

A checklist attached to the front of the bundle of documents to be taken to trial may remind the expert witness of all necessary arrangements.

Arriving at court

On arriving early at court, find out which court has been allocated for the case.

Look for the solicitor who has instructed you and confirm that you are present. Although in a clinical negligence case you are likely to have met the advocate in pre-trial conferences sometimes, due to the scheduling of cases, that advocate may be unavailable and another takes their place.

If this happens, the new advocate is likely to wish to go over the evidence with you. Be prepared for this to happen. If there has been a lot of activity in the days immediately prior to the trial resulting in new questions being raised within your field of expertise, or if circumstances require clarification of the evidence, the advocate will ask specific questions that need an almost immediate answer.

It is for this reason that access to all relevant papers including the complete textbooks used for the evidence are required in court. If you cannot give an answer to a question without consideration or consultation, then tell the advocate before the trial. He/she would much prefer a delayed but considered answer, supported by evidence, rather than a quick, incorrect response given because the expert felt under pressure.

Before the trial begins it is important for the legal and expert team to consider whether all witnesses are required to be present in court for the entire proceedings or only during parts of the trial.

As an expert in court you will have to listen to factual and expert evidence from the other party. This may be different under questioning from the version previously presented in the papers that were used in the preparation of your written evidence.

During the evidence from these witnesses a question may arise that you feel is relevant to be asked, or you may wish to make a comment if the evidence changes. Before trial, establish how the barrister wishes such communications to be made. Usually these are passed to him as a note (in legible writing).

Layout of the court (see Figure 5.2)

If you have not been called to court before, or if your experience is limited to a Crown Court, be aware that the layout of a civil court may be different. It is worthwhile asking the solicitor or the clerk of the court for a brief look at the layout of the court in order to assess the accoustics.

Procedure in court

During court proceedings the expert witnesses can sit in the court and usually sits with the solicitors in the row behind the advocates. The solicitor will have all the relevant bundles of documents available for reference, although the expert will also have their own copies. Witnesses of fact, which include any of the healthcare professionals involved in the case under question, cannot enter the court until called to give evidence and must remain outside the court after proceedings have commenced.

Should the expert wishes to enter or leave the court for any reason after the proceedings have begun they must acknowledge the judge with a bow as they enter or leave. In a complex trial with various experts, the legal team may only want some of them present for part of the trial. This will result in movement in the court. It is important that any movement of the expert does not detract from the solemnity of the proceedings and should be undertaken with care.

The role of the expert during the trial

While the major role of the expert in a trial is to give evidence on oath and to have that evidence examined by cross-examination, other functions performed by them during the proceedings.

Until the expert witness enters the witness box, they can be consulted by the party which has called them for confidential advice or information.

It is therefore vital that, when in the court, the expert listens to the evidence. There is no point in them being there unless they give their full attention to the proceedings. If a witness, either factual or expert, makes a statement that contradicts their previous evidence, the expert and the legal team should be aware of this. Ensure that the advocate is made aware by sending him or her a note. If the expert feels that there is a point in the evidence that is unclear, a note should be passed to the advocate requesting clarification. Remember that what may seem mundane and routine to another healthcare professional may not be clear even to a highly trained lawyer.

Remember, however, that it is the advocate who is conducting the case in court and while the information that the expert passes may, in their view, be important the advocate may choose to delay the use of the information.

It is also vital that the expert can prove if questioned later that they knew about a problem with the evidence. Any notes to counsel should therefore be made in duplicate, dated and timed and a copy kept.

If counsel feels that the note is important or if some evidence is unclear to him the counsel may turn round and directly ask the expert either to confirm a statement made by a witness or ask for clarification of a point.

Changes in the facts

One of the most important roles of the expert in court is to listen for any changes in the factual evidence. This is important as the opinion that the expert has given is based on the facts made available to them when preparing their report.

If, during the evidence, it becomes clear that the factual basis has changed and, as such, the opinion of the expert needs to be modified, this must be communicated to the legal team before the expert enters the witness box. If the change in the evidence is so great that all of the premises that your opinion relied on have changed and they now concord with the views of the opposing expert, then alerting the legal team early will allow them to decide if a settlement should be attempted.

Giving factual evidence

If the legal team defending the healthcare professional feel there is no evidence of sub-standard or negligent practice, the defendant healthcare professional will have to give evidence in court regarding the treatment they administered to the claimant patient.

When called to give evidence the healthcare professional should enter the court and the witness box. They should take the oath, using the holy book of their choice, or affirm using a firm, clear voice reading the words on the card slowly. This will allow any nervousness to lessen and also gives the speaker the chance to get used to hearing their own voice in the court accoustics.

The advocate will then take the healthcare professional through their evidence. The advocate will establish both the current occupation and the occupation of the healthcare professional at the time of the alleged incident of sub-standard care.

While the defendant practitioner may have made a statement regarding the episode, the only written evidence available to the healthcare professional now will be the clinical records.

Having taken the healthcare professional through their actions or omissions, the barrister will then invite the opposing counsel to cross-examine the witness.

This is the time that causes most fear in the witness. There are some simple guidelines which may lessen the anxiety.

Firstly, listen to the question and answer the question asked. The answer should be concise but should not be restricted if an explanation is required. Do not try and guess what the advocate is going to ask next, just answer one question at a time.

If you do not know the answer, say so. If the advocate quotes from the medical records, particularly a brief phrase, before answering the question, look at the relevant page and read the context of the phrase. If necessary, read out the whole passage before answering.

Do not be rushed into giving an answer if you feel that it requires some thought. If the advocate tries to hurry an answer, state politely that time is needed to consider the response.

Finally, direct all answers to the judge who will be recording both the questions and answers to make his or her judgement. Do not speak too quickly. If you do, the advocate or the judge is likely to ask you to slow down.

When cross-examination is complete, a re-examination of the points covered in cross-examination may be made by the original advocate. This can only be used to clarify points made previously and cannot be used to introduce new evidence.

If you have not given evidence before, or if you have had a bad experience of doing so, you may want to gain confidence by attending a courtroom skills training course (see **Appendix C**).

Giving expert evidence

Following the factual evidence, the expert evidence will be presented. At this point it is important for the expert to remember the change in their status and that their overriding duty is to the court.

Until the expert witness enters the witness box they have been advising one of the parties, in an impartial manner, on that party's case. Having entered the witness box, however, the expert witness cannot communicate with that party except in court until their evidence is completed.

What to take into the witness box

Although the expert will have their own copy of the report that was submitted to the court and all the textbooks and papers supporting their expert opinion, the expert witness should consider carefully before taking these into the witness box.

This is because there are likely to be annotations on the report. If this is taken into the witness box the report, including the annotations, will have to be disclosed to the other party if they so request.

It is even more important in this age of electronic communications that if the expert has an electronic copy of their evidence on their own portable computer, and they wish to take it into the witness box, no previous draft copies of the report or other copies of undisclosed letters to the legal team should be on the hard disk.

Taking the oath

Having entered the witness box the expert will take the oath in the same manner as a witness of fact.

Establishing expertise

In addition to establishing the name and occupation of the expert witness the court must be convinced that the person in the witness box is able to give expert evidence. It is therefore important for the advocate to establish the experience and qualifications of the expert witness and this is done after the identification process.

In most cases, counsel will ask the expert to give a brief resumé of their experience and expertise. This is not a time for false modesty and it is important for the credibility of the evidence that the healthcare professional later gives that, in the judge's mind, the expert witness is an appropriate person to give that evidence.

Evidence in chief

Having established the qualifications and expertise of the expert witness, the advocate will then examine the evidence that the witness wishes to present. As this is contained in the report that has been tendered in evidence, this will often be a very brief examination.

It will begin with the advocate asking if the report is the opinion of the healthcare professional. The advocate will then ask if there are any areas which the expert now wishes to change as a result of any evidence presented in court.

Sometimes the advocate may refer only to the vital points or occasionally may enquire about a weakness in the report. Answer all the questions honestly and fully, using the report as the basis of your evidence.

Cross-examination

The cross-examination of an expert witness has two functions. Firstly, to test the evidence and confirm that it is correct and secondly to confirm that the expert is indeed qualified to give the expert evidence.

A barrister may use many tactics to disconcert the expert but if the expert is aware of this he or she will be better able to deal with them.

Probably the most important advice when being cross-examined is that all answers should be directed to the judge. This is facilitated if, when entering the witness box, the expert stands facing the judge and then turns their upper body, keeping their feet still,towards the questioning advocate. Having listened to the question, the expert should turn back to face the judge and speak in that direction until the answer is completed before turning back to face the advocate for the next question.

In this way tactics like feigned disinterest or talking to the team seated behind the advocate during an answer, are less likely to be noticed by the witness and will be less off-putting.

Expect the advocate to question your credibility by asking about your present work and the relationship to the questions at issue in the case.

The expert may find that the advocate states that the expert is too young to have the experience or too old to be in active practice. Rarely are expert witnesses just at the "correct age".

The questioner may also use a technique of silence following an answer as though expecting some further answer. If you have completed your answer, stand quietly awaiting the next question. At other times, the exact opposite will occur, when the questioner will attempt to interrupt the answer. Be polite and ask the judge for permission to complete one answer before starting to answer another question.

If the advocate quotes from literature with which you are not familiar, then request time to study the original document to ensure that the suggested quotation is not taken out of context.

If you feel that any question requires some time to enable a considered answer, say so to the judge. Do not be intimidated into giving a quick answer which may be inaccurate, unhelpful to the judge and which you may later regret.

Remember that, as the expert, you have much more knowledge of your area than the advocate asking the questions. Use every opportunity when answering the questions to confirm your impartial views given in the report. If asked about a topic you have not considered and which is relevant, have the grace to accept that such an argument changes your opinion.

Finally, do not enter into point-scoring or an argument with the advocate. You are very likely to lose.

Re-examination

Having completed the cross-examination there is an opportunity for any areas previously touched on to be re-examined and clarified. If, during cross-examination the expert has been backed into a corner by the use of closed questions (a series of questions with yes/no answers) leading to an apparent change in the evidence, there is a chance that review of the evidence using an open question will enable a longer answer. Use this opportunity to its full extent.

In a complex case the period of examination, cross-examination and re-examination of an expert witness may span intervals of lunch and overnight.

The rules of evidence are clear. The witness may not have contact with the legal team during that whole period. While on all other days of the trial, lunch may be a corporate affair for the legal and expert team, when giving evidence, the expert should seek solitude over meal breaks and at the end of the day's proceedings.

If, during the process, there is a question that needs to be researched, the expert must carry out this research

without using the resources of the legal team. The
expert may, however, take advice from other
professionals not connected with the case.

Completing evidence

Having given the evidence and been cross-examined,
the expert can resume their seat in court behind the
legal team. Remember that any witness can be recalled
to give further evidence and is still under oath.

It is important that the expert does not relax at this
point. If there is other evidence still to be presented
this must be assimilated and should, the facts change
again, this must be communicated to the legal team.

Using the court as a learning experience

Following the conclusion of the case the expert should
have a debriefing session either on their own or with
the legal team. This should include all aspects of the
evidence given both in the reports prepared, the
conferences and meetings attended and the days in
court.

Listen to all the comments of the legal team; both the
solicitors and advocates. Analyse your own
performance. Look forward to using any changes in the
evidence, its presentation and the logistics of attending
trial for preparation of your evidence in the future.

12

Marketing an expert witness practice

Many healthcare professionals wrongly associate marketing with advertising, thinking that the two terms are interchangeable. Due to restrictions placed on advertising by regulating authorities, many practitioners do not involve themselves in marketing.

While there are still strict rules regarding advertising by healthcare professionals, these have been changed in recent years and the latest advice from the GMC regarding advertising is appended as an annex to this chapter.

The aim of this section is to examine briefly the whole area of marketing. This is much more than simple advertising and can be done even if the healthcare professional remains wary of formal advertising.

This section is however only an introduction to the subject of marketing and for those who wish to have a more in depth look at this whole area there are a list of titles included in the bibliography.

What then is marketing if it is not advertising?

Marketing is the concept of bringing a product or service to the attention of potential customers.

The major part of the marketing of any expert witness practice is the report which is written for the solicitor. In this book we have therefore discussed at length the structure and presentation of the report. Even if the opinion contained in the report is not what the solicitor wanted, a well presented and argued report shows the expert has taken care and is likely to do so again.

If the report is supportive of the case and is presented as evidence to the opposing side and in court, it will be seen by many other legal professionals who may provide further work in the future.

Like many professionals, the legal profession share information by both informal and formal means.

Many lawyers find recommendations informally about which expert witness to use and which to avoid.

All of the above methods are good for getting further work but, having secured the initial approach from a solicitor, many expert witnesses wonder how to get their first instruction.

While some may receive spontaneous inquires from the legal profession to their place of work this is uncommon outside personal injury instructions.

Gaining initial instructions

To gain initial instructions, expert witnesses need to seek out potential clients. The acceptable way of advertising approved by the GMC is to have oneself listed in the various expert witness directories (See Appendix D). Here, factual information conforming to the advertising standards agency code can be presented. This, however, is a passive form of marketing. An alternative method is to use your expertise either in written or oral form to present to potential clients. This may involve speaking to societies of lawyers or at conferences organized for the legal profession or writing articles in the legal press.

Even if not presenting at legal conferences, simply meeting lawyers in a social context can lead to useful introductions which may lead to future work.

Earlier in this book we commented on the need for the expert witness to be contactable either via a secretary or answering machine at all times.

In private medical practice it has been said that the qualities of a good private practitioner are ability, amiability and availability but not necessarily in that order. In the same way, the healthcare professional acting as an expert witness, if they ensure they are available, is likely to be used more often than the acknowledged authority who remains aloof and unapproachable.

In conclusion, even if the healthcare professional eschews formal advertising as a marketing tool, there are many other avenues that he or she can exploit to market their expert witness practice. The most visible and consistent tools are the quality of the reports they write and their attitude to those who instruct them.

Increasing your work

We recommend you attend a one day training course especially designed for expert witnesses e.g. "The Marketing Day" run by Bond Solon Training (See Appendix D). For a more detailed review of the subject, see "Marketing for Expert Witnesses" by C. Bond and J. Leppard, published by Bond Solon Publishing.

GENERAL MEDICAL COUNCIL

Protecting patients, guiding doctors

Providing Information About Your Services

(This guidance replaces the booklet Advertising)

1. If you publish or broadcast information about services you provide, the information must be factual and verifiable. It must be published in a way that conforms with the law and with the guidance issued by the Advertising Standards Authority. If you publish information about specialist services, you must still follow the guidance in paragraph 35 of Good Medical Practice.*

2. The information you publish must not make claims about the quality of your services nor include comparisons with the services provided by colleagues. It must not, in any way, offer guarantees of cures, nor exploit patients' vulnerability or lack of medical knowledge.

3. Information published about specialist services should include advice that patients cannot usually be seen or treated by specialists, either in the NHS or private practice, without an appropriate referral, usually from their general practitioner. Specialists should take all reasonable steps to ensure that a similar statement is included in any advertisement for specialist services issued by an organisation with which they are associated.

4. Information you publish about your services must not put pressure on people to use a service, for example by arousing ill-founded fear of future ill health. Similarly you must not advertise your services by visiting or telephoning prospective patients, either in person or through a deputy.

November 1997

---

*Specialists should not usually accept a patient without a referral from a general practitioner. If they do, they must inform the patient's general practitioner before providing treatment, unless the patient tells them not to or has no general practitioner. In these cases the specialist must be responsible for providing or arranging any aftercare which is necessary until another doctor agrees to take over.

(Good Medical Practice, paragraph 35).

Ideas for marketing an Expert Witness Practice

Write articles in both the professional press and in the legal journals about your special interest

Give talks to groups of lawyers either in their own practice or at conferences

Speak to the Local Law Society

Have your name in:
The Directories of Expert Witnesses e.g.
The Law Society Directory
The Register of Expert Witnesses

Join Professional Associations of Expert Witnesses e.g.

The Expert Witness Institute/The Academy of Experts

Have solicitors that have used your expertise place your name on legal group databases

APIL (Association of Personal Injury Lawyers)
FOIL (Federation of Insurance Lawyers)
AVMA (Action for Victims of Medical Accidents)
HCL (Health Care Lawyers)

Speak on issues of professional interest to the local and national media

Read "Marketing for Expert Witnesses" by C. Bond and J. Leppard, published by Bond Solon Publishing

See Appendix D for more details

13

Getting paid

Aims

This chapter will

- Show the sources of payment for medico legal work
- Demonstrate the use of terms of work
- Indicate the financial management needed in an expert witness practice
- Show how to get outstanding fees paid

Introduction

At every meeting of expert witnesses involved in medico-legal work, a constant topic of conversation is the payment of fees for work done. Many complain about the time taken to receive payment for even simple items of work performed.

The aim of this chapter is to give an understanding of the financial management of an expert witness practice.

What is the expert witness being paid for?

Some people, including the client of the instructing solicitor, think that the expert is being paid for the opinion that they reach or the expert is hired to further the case proposed by the client in the adversarial process.

As has been stressed before, the expert witness is an independent member of the team, giving advice. As such it is not the opinion that is being paid for but the time taken by the expert witness to reach that opinion and then to support that opinion throughout the legal process.

Who pays the expert witness?

The contract for payment of fees charged by the expert witness is usually between the expert witness and the instructing solicitor(s). Although the final payment of the expert witness is often from the side losing the court action (this may be as part of the costs of the case) there are various intermediate parties who will, directly or indirectly, pay the fees of the expert witness.

These include:

• the client themselves;

• the Legal Aid Board;

• legal expenses insurance firms;

• trade unions or professional associations;

• insurance companies;

• the solicitors in a "no win–no fee" case

In all these cases the expert witness's fee is "a disbursement" and should be met in accordance with the contract terms when the expert was instructed and within a reasonable time of the presentation of the invoice for the service rendered. In order to ensure this, however, the expert witness should agree terms for payment at the time of acccepting instructions. These should be agreed to *before* the expert witness starts work on his or her opinion.

Although the final bill may be met from another source, (once the final costs of the case are agreed or when assessed by the court), the contract is between the solicitor(s) and the expert witness. Therefore, the solicitor is liable for the fees of the expert witness and these fees should be met in accordance with the terms and conditions of the contract both parties agreed to. The expert witness should not have to wait outside the agreed terms and conditions of the contract with the solicitor even if the solicitor has not received these sums from either the client or the Legal Aid Board. However, if the solicitor has not received these funds, it will be difficult for many solicitors to pay the expert's fees.

It is for an expert to decide whether to work on "deferred fee terms" i.e to wait to be paid until the end of the case. There is no legal or professional objection to this.

When the solicitor agrees to the terms of the expert witness he or she becomes liable for the costs of that contract. This is irrespective of the amount of those costs that the solicitor's client may later be allowed at the conclusion of the case. The only exception to this would be if the solicitor indicates in the initial letter of instruction that the expert witness's fees will only be paid up to the level of the fees recovered on assessment by the court at the end of the case. If the solicitor imposes such a condition the expert witness must make a judgement as to whether they are willing to accept cases on such a basis. If the fees are reduced, the expert witness should be able to demonstrate the amount of work, (using time record sheets) involved in providing the opinion which would then be presented at the hearing to determine costs. This happens before a judge or a taxing master.

What should the expert witness charge?

Sometimes letters of instruction include the phrase 'we will be responsible for your reasonable fees'. The question of what is reasonable is difficult to quantify and will depend on the service being rendered and the person rendering the service.

The expert witness must endeavour to tread the line between being properly compensated for their time and experience and covering the costs associated with the administration of their practice, without pricing themselves out of the market, particularly as the court now has the power to control the amount of expert's fees which will be recoverable from the losing party.

What are the costs I need to consider?

Although each individual expert witness will have different costs in setting up and maintaining an expert witness practice, a checklist including most of the common costs is included at the end of this chapter. This will enable each individual to determine the approximate costs incurred in a practice. It is important for the expert witness to run their practice as a business. Otherwise there is a risk of not covering the costs incurred.

While some costs can be passed directly to the clients, there is a time element involved in the administration of the practice which needs to be included but cannot be charged directly to clients.

Having estimated the costs that the expert witness will incur over a time period, and then calculating the length of time you will work, a figure for the expenses involved based on an hourly rate can be estimated. Once costs are recovered, the additional amount the expert witness charges will be profit, assuming that the amount of work that was estimated can be achieved.

If less work is performed than the budget had anticipated at the beginning of the year, then the proportion of the fees needed to cover costs will be more and the amount left as profit for the expert witness will be less.

Having made this calculation, some may feel that the effort to achieve this figure may be too great and may decide not to continue with an expert witness practice.

What financial records does the expert witness need to keep?

The chapter on the organisation of an expert witness practice has already alluded to the need to keep financial records and the advisability for transparency in financial matters.

At the very least, this requires a separate business bank account for all of the financial transactions of the practice. Copies of all invoices must be retained and records of all monies paid must be kept. All receipts for expenses used in the practice must also be stored so that these can be claimed and, if challenged by the Inland Revenue, can be shown to have been spent on running the expert witness practice.

While a manual system can perform all of these functions adequately, a computerised accounts package will be able to do this and more. A computerised package can provide the expert with up to the minute reports on the state of the practice and, in addition, the amount of monies owed on outstanding invoices. Letters can automatically be created to chase late payment of fees, thus improving cash flow.

The legal aid fund

Some of the clients that a expert witness deals with have the funding of their case provided through the Legal Aid Board.

This is a publicly funded body where litigation costs are paid, in whole or part, by the state. These costs are approved either as a general cost, or a more specific cost, if an individual item costs a significant amount. Some initial letters of instruction asking for the expert witness to give an indication of the costs of the report are intended for review by the Legal Aid Board. This will allow the solicitor to obtain prior approval for this expenditure from the Legal Aid Board

The solicitor, having obtained the approximate fee for the report, applies to the Legal Aid Board for approval. Having received approval for a fee up to a specified maximum the solicitor can instruct the expert with a maximum fee provision. If the solicitor receives a fee note not exceeding the amount specified in the prior approval the Legal Aid Board will pay the solicitor. It is unlikely that this will be challenged when the costs are deliberated at taxation.

Most solicitors, however, do not send the entire bundle of medical or other notes when asking the expert for an indication of the fees. It can be difficult to determine the amount of work that a report will entail. Therefore, if too low a fee is tendered to the Legal Aid Board because the amount of work vastly exceeds that time, the expert is not guaranteed the fee. If the expert presents a fee within the maximum allowed the expert may then be working for free on the case.

It is therefore worthwhile including in the initial response to the solicitor a proviso that if the amount of work seen when the notes have arrived exceeds the estimate given, the expert will advise the solicitor of this before commencing work. This will allow the solicitor to return to the Legal Aid Board with a revised estimate for further approval.

Payments from the Legal Aid Board

Most requests from solicitors to the Legal Aid Board for disbursements, which include expert witness's fees, are handled speedily. The Legal Aid Board normally issues payment within 6 weeks and the cheque will be sent to the solicitor within that timeframe. Many solicitors will immediately forward the fee to the expert.

Therefore, expert witnesses should advise the solicitors regarding their fees and ask the solicitor to obtain prior approval. When the fee note is presented, payment should be made to the expert within two months.

How can the expert witness justify his or her fees?

Charging for expert witness work can either be based on an hourly rate or on a flat fee for a specific piece of work. Sometimes a combination of these calculation methods may be used by the same expert at different times. If the hourly rate is used as a basis for the fee then the expert has to determine the length of time a specific piece of work will take and then apply that hourly rate. While the hourly rate may not be questioned when it falls within a payment range similar experts charged by the amount of time taken by a specific expert to produce a piece of work may require some explanation.

To avoid this, it is worthwhile keeping a log of the time spent on each case. This can be sent to the solicitor if any dispute occurs regarding payment of the fees or at taxation. This can be a manual log or, if the practice is fully computerised, can be kept in a file on the hard disk of your computer. A copy of this log can either be sent with the fee note when it is prepared or can be made available at the end of the case should the fee be disputed.

How do I keep track of outstanding fees?

Outstanding fees should be regularly reviewed. If the accounts package used to compile the invoices is computerised, then a report of outstanding fees can be produced.

An individual letter reminding the solicitor of any outstanding fees can be prepared and a simple statement of the outstanding fees sent to the solicitor following a reasonable period of time since issue of the invoice.

How do I collect overdue fees?

Despite agreeing terms with the solicitor, there may be times when the expert witness's fees are not paid within the agreed time scale. This leaves the expert with a choice, either to chase the fees or to wait for the solicitor to pay.

Occasionally, there may be a single fee outstanding from a regular client when other fees presented after the outstanding fee have been paid. This may be an oversight, or the solicitor may not have received the report, through the vagaries of the postal system. In those cases a polite telephone call asking if the report has been received and pointing out that the fee remains outstanding may produce an apology that the fee has been overlooked and payment will be forthcoming.

Good relationships with clients should not be destroyed by aggressive debt collection letters to the practice without prior warning.

If there are single fees outstanding from non-regular clients then a simple reminder letter may produce the payment. Sometimes that initial contact does not produce the fees and if this is the case the expert witness has at least three options.

A Complaint to the Senior Partner

We have been advised by The Law Society that a sensible first step to recovery of expert's fees is to write to the senior partner of the firm concerned. Obviously, this will be of limited use in cases where you are already dealing with the senior partner.

Office for the Supervision of Solicitors

All solicitors are bound by a code of conduct which includes the payment of fees. It is a powerful argument that if the outstanding fees are not paid, the matter will be reported by the expert witness to the Office for the Supervision of Solicitors (the body which has succeeded the Solicitors Complaints Mechanism). The threat may be sufficient but if not, write to them (See Appendix D for address). This office will then investigate your complaint.

Sueing the solicitor

If the fees are not forthcoming the expert witness can sue the solicitor in the County Court for the outstanding fees or ask a debt collection agency to do so. At that time, any expenses and court fees will be charged to the solicitor. In addition to specific requests for payment, the expert witness should keep a general record of the time taken by specific firms to pay fees.

If new instructions are received from a firm where payment is unduly delayed the expert witness may decide not to accept instructions from that firm in future. The time involved in chasing debts reduces both the amount of time available for other work and the hourly rate charged for the work already done. The expert witness may also, if they take on the work, either add a premium to the fee to cover the expected delay in payment or ask the firm to pay for the work after it is prepared but before it is despatched to the solicitor.

By cultivating the firms that provide regular work and payment within the agreed time limit, the value of the work done and the cashflow are improved.

Paying tax

The aim of most expert witnesses is to make money from their expert practice. This is regarded by the Inland Revenue as self-employment income and as such, the tax due will be paid in lump sums. The expert witness involved in such activities should make provision for this by keeping back a percentage of the fees received in a deposit account to pay the tax demand. Otherwise, when the demand arrives, a loan from the bank may be needed to cover this expense. If payment of tax is not made in accordance with the rules then automatic penalties are imposed.

While the cost of a bank loan can be an expense of the practice, fines for late payment of tax are not.

Remember the expert witness is an expert in healthcare and not in accounting or the tax system. The early advice of an accountant when the expert witness is setting up their practice can not only save the costs of the advice in good planning, but will also free the expert witness from some of the financial activities, allowing them to concentrate on their area of expertise.

Also, speak to your tax office or accountant concerning the question of charging VAT on your reports.

Appendix A: Example Medical Report

XXXXXXXX *V* XXXXXXXX

Title of the action

XXXXXXXX

Court reference number

Final report of *your name* for the *name of the court*

Dated	:	*The date you sign your report and send it to the instructing solicitors.*
Specialist field	:	*Your specialist field*
On behalf of the Claimant/ Defendant	:	*The name of the party to the action*

This format is only a **suggestion**. It contains the main elements you will need to consider but you will need to create your own personal format that will depend on your specialist field and the particular case. This front page should be visible, preferably with transparent plastic sheet, although this is optional. Do not use comb binders. Use A4 good quality paper, hole punched for lever arch file with a slide binder. Find out from the solicitors who instruct you how many top copies are needed. The report must be addressed to the court.

Make sure you include your:
Name
Address
Telephone number
Fax number
Reference

Report of *your name*   page 2

Specialist field *your specialist field*

On behalf of *the Claimant/Defendant (or both) name of the party you have been instructed by*

Contents

This contents page is useful even if the report is short. In longer reports, the contents page may need to be more detailed so the reader can easily find their way around the report.

Report of *your name*   **page 3**

Specialist field *your specialist field*

On behalf of *the Claimant/Defendant (or both) name of the party you have been instructed by*

Report

1   Introduction

1.01   The writer

I am *your full name*. My specialist field is *your specialist field and give a short summary of the most important qualifications and experience relevant to the case. No more than three lines.* Full details of my qualifications and experience entitling me to give expert opinion evidence are in appendix 1. *It is necessary to have these full details as you may be cross examined on them.*

1.02   Summary of the case

The case concerns *give a short outline of the case.* There is a chronology of the key events in appendix 5. I have been instructed to *say briefly what you have been asked to do.*

1.03   Summary of my conclusions

This report will show that in my professional opinion *give your conclusion. It is good practice to put an executive summary at the beginning so that the reader knows the direction of your analysis.*

1.04   The parties involved

Those involved in the case are as follows:

List the people and organisations you refer to in your report with a short description of each. This can be very useful for a judge.

1.05   Medical terms and explanations

I have indicated any medical terms in **bold type**. I have defined these terms when first used and included them in a glossary in appendix 6. I have also included in appendix 3 extracts of published works I refer to in my report and in appendix 4 there are diagrams and photographs to assist in the understanding of the case.

Report of *your name*   **page 4**

Specialist field *your specialist field*

On behalf of *the Claimant/Defendant name of the party you have been instructed by*

2   The issues to be addressed

2.01   Set out the issues you will address in your report. Number each issue as you
          will refer to each in your opinion in paragraph 4. Do not give your opinion
          here. Distinguish liability and quantum.

Report of *your name*   **page 5**

Specialist field *your specialist field*

On behalf of *the Claimant/Defendant name of the party you have been instructed by*

---

3   My investigation of the facts

This section establishes the foundation of fact upon which you will base your opinion. The starting point is 'I do not know, but let me see what the facts are'. Set out the facts of the case as you see them. Identify the source of these facts. You must distinguish fact from opinion. Also distinguish facts you have been told and those you personally observed. This paragraph is purely factual. Paragraph 4 will deal with your opinion.

3.01   Documents

Identify the important documents for the judge. Remember appendix 2 contains a list of the documents you have considered with copies of the really important documents. Medical records are particularly important.

3.02   Interview and medical examination

Give details of any interview and examination you did. Give dates and times. Say if anyone else was present.

3.03   Research

Give details of any research papers you considered. Remember appendix 3 contains a list of published works you refer to and has copy extracts.

3.04   Experiments

Give details of any experiments you did to prepare for the report.

Report of *your name*   **page 6**

Specialist field *your specialist field*

On behalf of *the Claimant/Defendant name of the party you have been instructed by*

Things you may need to include will depend on the particular case. This alphabetical list gives some of the more important topics. You will need to order them logically.

Before and after picture

Equipment used and need

Immediate effects of the injury

Incident, description

Pain and suffering, past and current

Patient information, include name, date of birth, marital status, dependants occupation

Place, size, plans

Precisely what injuries the patient suffered

Present complaints

Previous medical history

Procedures

Protocol

Qualifications and employment facts

Records

Routine

Set the scene

Special training for the task

Staffing

Training

Be careful with any statement of the patient as to how the incident happened. Distinguish what you were told and what you noticed yourself. Be prepared to be cross examined on your recollection.

4   My opinion

Go through each issue identified in paragraph 2, link these to the facts from paragraph 3 and then give your reasoned argument for the opinion you come to. Facts, analysis then argued conclusion. Remember the reader of your report does not have your knowledge and expertise. He needs to have your thinking <u>explained</u>. Avoid using the word negligence as this is a legal term. Let the judge make the decision, so just give your professional opinion. Do not give a legal opinion.

The CPR require that where there is a range of opinion on the matters dealt with in your report, you summarise the range of opinion and give your reasons for your opinion.

A possible format is
* Careful analysis of the facts
* Medical explanation using lots of illustrations
* Relate the case to your medical explanation

In medical negligence cases
* Remember the **'Bolam'** test: 'A doctor is not guilty of negligence if he has acted in accordance with a practice accepted as proper by a responsible body of medical men skilled in that particular art … a doctor is not negligent, if he is acting in accordance with such a practice, merely because there is a body of opinion that takes a contrary view.' Breach of duty: 'The test is the standard of the ordinary skilled man exercising and professing to have that special skill. A man need not possess the highest expert skill; it is well established law that it is sufficient if he exercises the ordinary skill of an ordinary competent man exercising that particular art.'

Personal injury
Includes any disease of a person's physical or mental condition.

Causation
'But for …' test
* What happened? Historical fact.
* What would have happened but for the matter complained of? Hypothetical fact.
* What is the difference?

Report of *your name*   **page 8**

Specialist field *your specialist field*

On behalf of *the Claimant/Defendant name of the party you have been instructed by*

Watch for
* The effect of a medical intervention on an underlying disease.
* There may be several concurrent or sequential conditions contributing to the injury.

Under quantum you may include:

Comments on other expert's reports

Future employment prospects (*remember you are not an employment expert*)

Handicap permanent or temporary

Loss of life expectancy

Other experts needed

Prognosis

Declaration and Statement of truth

Signature.. Date................................

N.B.: Do not forget to sign and date your report!

Report of *your name*   page 9

Specialist field *your specialist field*

On behalf of *the Claimant/Defendant name of the party you have been instructed by*

Appendix 1

Details of my qualifications and experience

This is the front sheet for the contents of the appendix. Have a separate front sheet for each appendix.

Appendix 7

Declaration taken from the Expert Witness Institute's draft Declaration

1. I understand that my overriding duty is to the court, both in preparing reports and in giving oral evidence.
2. I have set out in my report what I understand from those instructing me to be the questions in respect of which my opinions as an expert are required. [1]
3. I have done my best, in preparing this report, to be accurate and complete. I have mentioned all matters which I regard as relevant to the opinions I expressed. All of the matters on which I have expressed an opinion lie within my field of expertise.
4. I have drawn to the attention of the court all matters, of which I am aware, which might adversely affect my opinion.
5. Wherever I have no personal knowledge, I have indicated the source of factual information.
6. I have not included anything in this report which has been suggested to me by anyone, including lawyers instructing me, without forming my own independent view of the matter.
7. Where, in my view, there is a range of reasonable opinion, I have indicated the extent of that range in my report.
8. At the time of signing the report I consider it to be complete and accurate. I will notify those instructing me if, for any reason, I subsequently consider that the report requires any correction or qualification.
9. I understand that this report will be the evidence that I will give under oath, subject to any correction or qualification I may make before swearing to its veracity.
10. I have attached to this report a summary of my instructions.

I believe that the facts I have stated in this report are true and that the opinions I have expressed are correct.

Note
1. The point of this is to ensure that the expert is directing his/her opinion to the relevant issues. Experience shows that unless this is done, much time can be wasted on the wrong question.

Guidance notes
1. *The declaration should be considered carefully by the expert. Signing it is not a routine matter. If any part of it requires modification accordingly. Thus in some cases, an expert's instructions may limit the scope of the report and paragraph 2 may require modification accordingly.*
2. *The declaration is appropriate only for **civil** cases.*
3. *The declaration is not about ethics, but about responsibilities.*
4. *The declaration is only appropriately associated with the **final report** for exchange.*
5. *The declaration should be served as an appendix to the final report.*

page 11

Here is a check list to use when you have completed your report.

yes ✔	no ✔	
☐	☐	A4 good quality paper, hole punched for lever arch file
☐	☐	Chronology
☐	☐	Clear headings
☐	☐	Contents page
☐	☐	Covering letter and invoice
☐	☐	Dated
☐	☐	Double spaced or space and a half
☐	☐	Expressed in the first person
☐	☐	Front sheet
☐	☐	Glossary
☐	☐	Graphics
☐	☐	Headers on each page
☐	☐	Margins wide enough for written comments
☐	☐	Pages numbered
☐	☐	Paragraphs numbered
☐	☐	Publications dated and precede incident date (if appropriate)
☐	☐	Short sentences and paragraphs?
☐	☐	Summary of instructions
☐	☐	Declaration, Statement of truth signed
☐	☐	Synopsis

Review the following pointers:

Accurate?

Clear conclusion?

Fact and opinion clearly separated?

Good use of appendices?

How concise is the report?

How clearly are the issues identified?

How clear is the language for a non expert to read?

How logical is the report?

How far does the report stand alone i.e. contains everything that the judge would need?

How well are the qualifications and experience set out?

Quality of paper?

Quality of printing?

EASY for judges and lawyers to use!

Appendix B

DRAFT CODE OF GUIDANCE FOR EXPERTS UNDER THE CIVIL PROCEDURE RULES 1998 (CPR)

The Code of Guidance, as and when approved by the Vice-Chancellor, will be converted into a Practice Direction; as such, it will have the same status as any other Practice Direction made under CPR. This will be subject to amendment from time to time as the case law on Part 35 develops.

Preamble

This code of guidance is designed to help those who instruct experts (and those instructed) in all cases where CPR applies. It is intended to facilitate better communication and dealings both between the expert and the instructing party and between the parties. Assistance from an expert may be needed at various stages of a dispute and for different purposes, the expert performing a different role in each of these respects. The duty to the court and the duty to act in the best interests of the party instructing the expert (including the expert's advisory role) will differ depending upon the context. When preparing a report for use in evidence at court or when giving oral evidence, however, the expert has an overriding duty to the court. The expert remains under a duty to comply with any relevant professional code of ethics. The court is likely to take into account adherence to the Code of Guidance in exercising its discretion as to costs.

PART I: EXPERTS

Advice and who Report   1   For the purpose of this Code a distinction is drawn between: experts

      a. are instructed to act solely in an advisory capacity(*advice*); and
      b. asked to give or prepare evidence for the purpose of court proceedings *report*).

Experts who are instructed by solicitors on behalf of their client to provide advice owe a duty to the client; in the event that the matter proceeds to litigation the expert's overriding duty is to the court.

Appointment   2   Those intending to appoint experts ought to consider whether the appointment is appropriate, taking account of the principles set out in Parts 1 and 35 of CPR, for which the following factors ought to be considered:

whether

    a. evidence will be necessary from an expert witness to prove facts in issue

    b. opinion evidence from an expert is relevant and will be helpful in resolving the dispute;

    c. sub paragraphs a) and b) can be achieved by the appointment of a single joint expert;

    d. the expert has the experience, expertise and training appropriate to the value, complexity and importance of the case; and

    e. the expert will be able to produce a report within a reasonable time of instruction and at a cost proportionate to the matters in issue.

Terms of appointment

3. Terms of appointment should be agreed at the outset and should include:

    a. the basis of the expert's charges (either daily or hourly rates and an estimate of the time likely to be required, or a fee for the services);

    b. any travelling expenses and other disbursements;

    c. rates for attendance at court and provisions for payment on late notice of cancellation of a court hearing;

    d. time for delivery of report;

    e. time for making payment; and

    f. whether fees are to be paid by a third party.

Payment

4. Payments contingent upon the nature of the expert evidence given in legal proceedings, or upon the outcome of a case, must not be offered or accepted, because to do otherwise might contravene the expert's overriding duty to the court.

Instructions

5. Experts should be kept informed regularly about any deadlines for the preparation of their *advice or reports*, and about any timetable for proceedings.

6. Those instructing experts should ensure that they give clear instruction, including the following:

    a. basic information, such as names, addresses, telephone numbers, dates of birth and dates of incidents;

    b. the nature and extent of expertise which is called for;

    c. the purpose of requesting the *advice or report*, a description of the matter to be investigated, the principle, known issues and the identity of all parties;

    d. the statement of case (if any), those documents which form part of standard disclosure and witness statements which are relevant to the *advice or report*;

    e. where proceedings have not been started, whether proceedings are being contemplated and, if so, whether the expert is asked only for *advice*; and

    f. where proceedings have been started, the date of any hearing and in which court and to which track they have been allocated.

7. Experts who do not receive such clear instructions should request them and withdraw from the case unless such instructions are received.

8. Those instructing experts should consider whether it is necessary to consult experts in respect of those parts of the statement of case to which their expertise is relevant.

9. Experts must neither express an opinion outside the scope of their field of expertise, nor accept any instructions to do so.

Experts' duties

10. It is the duty of experts:

    a. i) in the case of *advice*, to explain to those instructing them both the strengths and weaknesses of the parties'cases;
    ii) to explain in their *reports* to the court the range of opinion as required by Practice Direction 1.2(5)
    b. to agree a time limit with those instructing experts and to give notice of any delay beyond the deadline as soon as possible;
    c. to maintain professional objectivity at all times;
    d. when giving or preparing a *report*, or giving evidence either orally or in writing, to assist the court; and
    e. to supply references in respect of relevant literature or any other material which might assist the court in deciding the case.

11. As and when experts' *advice* becomes a *report*, an opportunity must be afforded to the experts to amend their advice.

Content of *Report*

12. In providing a *report* experts:

    a. must address it to the court and not to the parties;
    b. must express any qualification of, or reservation to their opinion
    c. if such opinion was not formed independently, should make it clear from whom the opinion was adopted;
    d. must not be asked to, and must not amend, expand or alter any part of the *report* in a manner which distorts the experts' true opinion; but
    e. may be invited to amend, or expand a *report* to ensure accuracy and internal consistency, completeness and clarity.

Information

13. All experts' *advice* and *reports* should contain the following information, except that sub-paragraphs (f) – (h) inclusive apply only to *reports*:

    a. academic and professional qualifications;
    b. a statement of the source of instructions and the purpose of the *advice or report*;
    c. a chronology of the relevant events;
    d. a statement of the methodology used, in particular what laboratory or other tests (if any) were employed, by whom and under whose supervision;
    e. details of the documents or any other evidence upon which any aspects of the *advice or report* is based;

    and in the case of experts' *reports only*:

    f. a statement setting out the substance of all instructions (whether written or oral). The statement should summarise the facts and instructions given to the expert which are material to the opinions expressed in the report or upon which those opinions are based;

g. a declaration that the *report* has been prepared in accordance with this Code; and

h. a statement of truth,as required by Part 35.

Fact and Opinion	14. In addressing questions of fact and opinion in any *advice or report* experts should keep the two separate and discrete.

Factual evidence
15. Where there is conflict of factual evidence, experts:

a. should not express a view in favour of one or other competing sets of facts, unless, because of their particular learning and experience, they perceive one set of facts as being improbable or less probable, in which case they may express that view, and should give reasons;

b. should express separate opinions on every set of facts in issue.

Procedure
16. Following completion of the *report*, experts should be:

a. advised whether, and if so when, the *report* has been disclosed to the other side;

b. given the opportunity to consider and comment upon other *reports* which deal with the same issues; and

c. be kept informed of the progress of the action, including any amendments to the stated case relevant to the expert's opinion.

Questions *report* for experts
17. A party may put questions to another party's expert about that expert's

a. In accordance with Rule 35.6;

b. Within the time limits prescribed within Rule 35.6 (2) and Practice Direction 4.1; or

c. Where the expert has sought directions from the court under Rule 35.14

Any such questions should be answered within 28 days.

Conferences and discussions
18. The parties and their lawyers should seek to reach agreement of, and consider taking steps to clarify, the issues by way of:

a. conference or discussion with experts; and /or

b. discussion between experts for opposing parties in order to identify

i   the extent of the agreement between experts;

ii   the points of disagreement and the reasons for disagreement;

iii action, if any, which may be taken to resolve the outstanding points of disagreement; and

iv any issues not raised in the agenda for discussion and the extent to which these issues may be agreed.

19. The parties, their lawyers and experts should co-operate to produce concise agendas for any discussion between experts, which should, so far as possible:

a. be circulated 28 days before the date fixed for the discussion;

b. be agreed 7 days before the date fixed for the discussion;

c. consist of questions which are clearly stated and apply, where necessary the correct legal test;

    d. consist of questions which are closed in their nature, that is to say capable of being answered "yes" or "no"; and

    e. consist of questions such as to enable the experts to state their agreement or the reasons for their disagreement with each other.

20. The discussion will take place preferably face to face except in small claims and fast track cases. Lawyers for the parties will not usually be present at such discussions.

21. If there has been a discussion, a statement of the areas of agreement and disagreement should be prepared and agreed promptly between the experts, usually before the discussion is concluded. This statement may have to be produced to the court, but shall not be binding on the parties.

22. Those instructing experts must not give, and experts must not accept, instructions not to reach agreement at such discussions on areas within the competence of experts.

Attendance at trial

23. The use of available audio-visual facilities should be relied upon to avoid unnecessary attendance at court.

24. Those instructing experts should inform them whether attendance at trial will be required, and if so inform them of the date and venue fixed for hearing of the case. In applying to fix dates for the trial, those instructing experts should accommodate, as far as possible, the convenience of experts.

25. Experts must take all steps to ensure availability to attend court, if and when required, but should be alerted to the fact that a solicitor may need to serve a witness summons in the event of difficulties.

PART II: SINGLE JOINT EXPERT

26. Where parties have agreed to, or the court directs the joint instruction of a single joint expert:

    a. parties should wherever possible agree the instructions be given jointly, failing which separate instructions shall be given to the single joint expert and a copy be sent to the other party;

    b. all instructions shall be given in writing;

    c. paragraphs 6 and 7 of Part I above shall apply.

27. The single joint Expert

    a. should provide a *report* which complies strictly with the provisions relating to *reports* of the parties; experts under Paragraphs 12 and 13 of Part I above; and

    b. may be questioned and shall provide answers in accordance with paragraph 17 above.

PART III: ASSESSORS

Appointment   28. The following guidance is subject to section 70(1) of the Supreme Court Act 1981and section 63 of the County Courts Act 1984 respectively, and Article 6(1) of the European Convention on Human Rights, as it appears in schedule I to the Human Rights Act 1998.

29. A party may at the outset of the proceedings, if it thinks it would be useful for the court to do so, apply to the court for the appointment of a person of skill and experience to provide an expert opinion on any matter to which the proceedings relate, either in place of the parties' experts or in addition to experts.

30. Where the parties' experts engage in discussions pursuant to Rule 35.12 or paragraphs 18 (b) and 19 above, the parties may request the court to appoint an assessor to preside over the discussions.

31. In requesting the court to appoint an assessor(s) the requesting party should indicate:

  a. the matter(s) in respect of which assistance of an assessor will be sought;
  b. the name(s) of the proposed assessor(s); and
  c. the precise area(s) of expertise to be covered by the assessor(s).

32. Any party requesting the court to appoint an assessor, for the purpose of assisting the court to decide any matter which involves expert opinion, shall notify other parties in writing of such request. Other parties so notified may submit to the court within 14 days their views on the proposed appointment.

Role and function of the assessor   33. Assessor(s) shall:

  a. provide a written report to court; and
  b. circulate it to the parties.

Parties may question the assessor(s) in accordance with CPR Part 35.6 the assessor(s) to file answers with the court and the parties.

34. Where there remains a conflict of expert opinion between the assessor(s) and the parties' experts, any party may apply to the court for permission to call experts to give oral evidence.

Appendix C: Extracts from The new Civil Procedure Rules and Practice Direction

Part 35 – Experts and Assessors

General duty of the court and the parties

35.1.   Expert evidence shall be restricted to that which is reasonably required to resolve the proceedings

Interpretation

35.2.   A reference to an 'expert' in this Part is a reference to an expert who has been instructed to give or prepare evidence for the purpose of court proceedings

Experts – overriding duty to the court

35.3   1.   It is the duty of an expert to help the court on the matters within his expertise

   2.   This duty overrides any obligation to the person from whom he has received

Court's power to restrict expert evidence

35.4   1.   No party may call an expert of put in evidence an expert's report without the court's permission

   2.   When a party applies for permission under this rule he must identify –

      a.   The field in which he wishes to rely on expert evidence and
      b.   Where practicable the expert in that field on whose evidence he wishes to rely.

   3.   If permission is granted under this rule it shall be in relation only to the expert named or the field identified under paragraph 2.

   4.   The court may limit the amount of the expert's fees and expenses that the party who wishes to rely on the expert may recover from any other party.

General requirement for expert evidence to be given in a written report

35.5 1. Expert evidence is to be given in a written report unless the court directs otherwise.

2. If a claim is on the fast track, the court will not direct an expert to attend a hearing unless it is necessary to do so in the interests of justice

Written questions to experts

35.6 1. A party may put to –

a. an expert instructed by another party; or
b. a single joint expert appointed under rule 35.7
    written questions about his report

2. Written questions under paragraph 1

a. may be put once only;
b. must be put within 28 days of service of the expert's report; and
c. must be put for the purpose only of clarification of the report;
    unless in any case,
i. the court gives permission; or
ii. the other party agrees.

3. An expert's answers to questions put in accordance with paragraph 1 shall be treated as part of the expert's report.

4. Where

a. a party has put in a written question to an expert instructed by another party in accordance with this rule; and
b. the expert does not answer that question,
    the court may make one or both of the following orders in relation to the party who instructed the expert
i. that the party may rely on the evidence of that expert; or
ii. that the party may not recover the fees and expenses of that expert from any other party

Court's power to direct that evidence is to be given by a single joint expert

35.7 1. Where two or more parties wish to submit expert evidence on a particular issue, the court may direct
    that the evidence on that issue is to be given by one expert only.

2. The parties wishing to submit the expert evidence are called 'the instructing parties'.

3. Where the instructing parties cannot agree who should be the expert, the court may;

a. Select the expert from a list of experts prepared or identified by the instructing parties; or
b. Direct that the expert be selected from such a manner as the court may direct.

Instructions to a single joint expert

35.8 1. Where the court gives a direction under rule 35.7 for a single joint expert to be used, each instructing party may give instructions to the expert

2. When an instructing party gives instructions to the expert he must, at the same time, send a copy of the instructions to the other instructing parties.

3. The court may give directions about the arrangements for –

    a. The payment of the expert's fees and expenses; and

    b. Any inspections, examinations or experiments which the expert wishes to carry out

4. The court may, before an expert is instructed –

    a. Limit the amount that can be paid by way of fees and expenses to the expert; and

    b. Direct that the instructing parties pay that amount into court

5. Unless the court otherwise directs, the instructing parties are jointly and severally liable for the payment of the expert's fees and expenses.

Power of court to direct a party to provide information

35.9. Where a party has access to information which is not reasonably available to the other party, the court may direct the party who has access to the information to –

    a. prepare and file a document recording the information; and

    b. serve a copy of that document on the other party

Contents of report

35.10 1. An expert's report must comply with the requirements set out in the relevant practice direction.

    2. At the end of an expert's report there must be a statement that

    a. The expert understands his duty to the court; and

    b. He has complied with that duty

    3. The expert's report must state the substance of all material instructions, whether written or oral, on the basis of which the report was written

    4. The instructions referred to in paragraph (3) shall not be privileged against disclosure but the court will not, in relation to those instructions –

    a. Order disclosure of any specific document; or

    b. Permit any questioning in court, other than by the party who instructed the expert, unless it is satisfied that there are reasonable ground to consider the statement of instructions given under paragraph (3) to be inaccurate or incomplete.

Use by one party of expert's report disclosed by another

35.11 Where a party has disclosed an expert's report, any party may use that expert's report as evidence at the trial.

Discussions between experts

35.12 1. The court may, at any stage, direct a discussion between experts for the purpose of requiring the experts to –

    a. Identify the issues in the proceedings; and

    b. Where possible, reach agreement on an issue

    2. The court may specify the issues which the experts must discuss

3.   The court may direct that following a discussion between the experts they must prepare a statement for the court showing –
     a.   those issues on which they agree; and
     b.   those issues on which they disagree and a summary of their reasons for disagreeing

4.   The content of the discussion between the experts shall not be referred to at the trial unless the parties agree.

5.   Where experts reach agreement on an issue during their discussions, the agreement shall not bind the parties unless the parties expressly agree to be bound by the agreement.

Consequence of failure to disclose expert's report

35.13   A party who fails to disclose an expert's report may not use the report at the trial or call the expert to give evidence orally unless the court gives permission.

Expert's right to ask court for directions

35.14   1.   An expert may file a written request for directions to assist him in carrying out his functions as an expert

2.   An expert may request directions under paragraph 1 without giving notice to any party.

3.   The court when it gives directions, may also direct that a party be served with one or both of –

     a.   A copy of the directions; and
     b.   A copy of the request for directions.

Assessors

35.15   1.   This rule applies where the court appoints one or more persons (an 'assessor') under section 70 of the Supreme Court Act 1981 (a) or section 63 of the County Courts Act 1984 (b)

2.   The assessor shall assist the court in dealing with a matter in which the assessor has skill and experience

3.   An assessor shall take such part in the proceedings as the court may direct and in particular the court may –

     a.   Direct the assessor to prepare a report for the court on any matter at issue in the proceedings; and
     b.   Direct the assessor to attend the whole or any part of the trial to advise the court on any such matter.

4.   If the assessor prepares a report for the court before the trial has begun –

     a.   The court will send a copy to each of the parties; and
     b.   The parties may use it at trial

5.   The remuneration to be paid to the assessor for his services shall be determined by the court and shall form part of the costs of the proceedings

6.   The court may order any party to deposit in the court office a specified sum in respect of the assessor's fees and where it does so the assessor will not be asked to act until the sum has been deposited

7.   Paragraphs 5 and 6 do not apply where the remuneration of the assessor is to be paid out of money provided by Parliament

Practice Direction – Experts and Assessors, Part 35

Part 35 is intended to limit the use of oral expert evidence to that which is reasonably required. In addition, where possible, matters requiring expert evidence should be dealt with by a single expert. Permission of the court is always required either to call an expert or to put an expert's report in evidence.

Form and Content of expert's reports

1.1.   An expert's report should be addressed to the court and not to the party from whom the expert has received his instructions.

1.2.   An expert's report must;

(1)give details of the expert's qualifications,
(2)give details of any literature or other material, which the expert has relied on in making the report
(3)say who carried out any test or experiment which the expert has used for the report and whether or not the test or experiment has been carried out under expert's supervision,
(4)give the qualifications of the person who carried out any such test or experiment, and
(5)where there is a range of opinion on the matters dealt with in the report –

(i)summarise the range of opinion, and
(ii)give reasons for his own opinion,

(6)contain a summary of the conclusions reached
(7)contain a statement that the expert understands his duty to the court and has complied with that duty (rule 35.10 (2)), and
(8)contain a statement setting out the substance of all material instructions (whether write or oral). The statement should summarise the facts and instructions given to the expert which are material to the opinions expressed in the report or upon which those opinions are based (rule 35.10 (3))

1.3.   An expert's report must be verified by a statement of truth as well as containing the statements required in paragraph 1.2 (7) and (8)

1.4.   The form of the statement of truth is as follows: " I believe that the facts I have stated in this report are true and that the opinions I have expressed are correct."

1.5.   Attention is drawn to rule 32.14 which sets out the consequences of verifying a document containing a false statement without an honest belief in its truth (For information about statements of truth see Part 22 and the practice direction which supplements it)

1.6.   In addition, an expert's report should comply with the requirements of any approved expert's protocol.

Information

2   Where the court makes an order under rule 35.9 (i.e where one party has access to information not reasonably available to the other party), the document to be prepared recording the information should set out sufficient details of any facts, test or experiments which constitute the information to enable an assessment and understanding of the significance of the information to be made and obtained.

Instructions

3   The instructions referred to in paragraph 1.2 (8) will not be protected by privilege (see rule 25.10(4). But cross-examination of the expert on the contents of his instructions will not be allowed unless the court permits it (or unless the party who gave the instructions consents to it). Before it gives permission the court must be satisfied that there are reasonable grounds to consider that the statement in the report of the substance of the instructions is inaccurate or incomplete. If the court is so satisfied, it will allow the cross-examination where it appears to be in the interests of justice to do so.

Questions to experts

4.1.   Questions asked for the purpose of clarifying the expert's report (see rule 35.6) should be put, in writing, to the expert not later than 28 days after receipt of the expert's report. (See paragraphs 1.2 to 1.5 above as to verification.)

4.2.   Where such a party sends a written question or questions direct to an expert and the other party is represented by solicitors, a copy of the questions should. At the same time, be sent to those solicitors.

Single expert:

5.   Where one court has directed that the evidence on a particular issue is to be given by one expert only (rule 35.7) but there are a number of disciplines relevant to that issue, a leading expert in the dominant discipline should be identified as the single expert. He should prepare the general part of the report and be responsible for annexing or incorporating the contents of any reports from experts in other disciplines.

Assessors

6.1.   An assessor may be appointed to assist the court under rule 35.15. Not less than 21 days before making any such appointment, the court will notify each party in writing of the name of the proposed assessor, of the matter in respect of which the assistance of the assessor will be sought and of the qualifications of the assessor to give that assistance.

6.2.   Where any person has been proposed for appointment as an assessor, objection to him, either personally or in respect of his qualification, may be taken, by any party.

6.3.   Any such objection must be made in writing and filed with the court within 7 days of receipt of the notification referred to is paragraph 6.1 and will be taken into account by the court in deciding whether or not to make the appointment (s 63 (5) County Courts Act 1984)

6.4.   Copies of any report prepared by the assessor will be sent to each of the parties but the assessor will not give oral evidence or be open to cross-examination or questioning.

Appendix D
Useful addresses

The Law Society
113 Chancery Lane
London WC2A 1SX
Tel: 0171 242 1222

Bond Solon Training & Publishing
13 Britton Street
London EC1M 5SX
Tel: 020 7253 7053
Fax: 020 7253 7051
E-mail: witness@bondsolon.bdx.co.uk
www.bondsolon.com

*Advice given on expert witness training &
conferences and can provide example of
experts' fees. Can also provide books for expert
witnesses on marketing and giving evidence in
court.*

**The UK Register of Expert
Witnesses**
JS Publications
Goodwin House
Willie Smith Road
Newmarket
Suffolk CB8 7SQ
Tel: 01638 561590

**The Law Society Directory of
Expert Witnesses**
Published by Sweet & Maxwell
100 Avenue Road
Swiss Cottage
London NW3 3PF
Tel: 0800 289618
Fax: 0171 449 1144

The Expert Witness Institute
Newspaper House
8–16 Great New Street
London EC4A 3BN
Tel: 0171 583 5454
Fax: 0171 583 5450

**Action for Victims of Medical
Accidents (AVMA)**
44 High Street
Croydon
Surrey CR0 1YB
Tel: 0181 686 6900
Fax: 0181 667 9065

Association of Personal Injury Lawyers
33 Pilcher Gate
Nottingham NG1 1QE
Tel: 0115 958 0585
Fax: 0115 958 0885

Office for the Supervision of Solicitors
Victoria Court
8 Dormer Place
Royal Leamington Spa
Warwickshire CV32 5AE
Tel: 01926 820082/3
Fax: 01926 431435

Avebury Computing Ltd
Clevedon, Brays Lane
Hyde Heath
Amersham
Buckinghamshire HP6 5RU
Tel/Fax: 01494 776142

Sells sample expert medical reports on disk.

Motor Accidents Solicitors Association
Bridge House
48–52 Baldwin Street
Bristol BS1 1QD
Tel: 0117 929 2560

Software Suppliers
Winslow New Ltd
29 Stanbury Close
Bosham
West Sussex
PO18 8NS
Tel: 01243 575818
E-mail: ceta@globalnet.co.uk

Index